Decades of Uplifting Short Stories for Seniors

1st Edition
The author is represented by: Keep your mind young
Address: Unser Frau 169, 39020 Schnals, Italy
Contact: wegamedia@gmail.com
Year of Publication: 2023
ISBN: 9791281260047
Head of Printing: Amazon KDP Publishing

50s 60s 70s 80s 90s

Contents

Introduction

Looking back over the past decades and reminiscing about things we remember is something everyone enjoys doing. Whether you came of age in the 1950s or are a product of the 1990s, remembering those decades is fun, enjoyable, and the perfect way to connect with others. Think about how much you enjoy talking to your grandchildren about past events they are learning about in history, especially when you can share your own experiences too.

This book contains 100 uplifting and positive stories, all related to specific decades. The stories bring fashion, current events, political climate, and more to life. Written from the viewpoint of someone who lived through the events, each level has an inspiring message and theme. Narratives are divided into decades, making reconnecting with your favorite era easier. They may also bring back memories that you have long forgotten.

Suppose you are looking for short tales that promote health, sparking long-forgotten memories and creating connections between your generation and the next. In that case, these stories are exactly what you want. Every narrative is uplifting, inspiring, and sometimes humorous, bringing the reader comfort, joy, and hope. They also provide a unique perspective on aging, making them perfect for those who lived through these decades and for younger people who may want an inside view of what it was like to live during those years.

Although based on historical facts, these are not strictly facts regurgitated in a new way. Instead, they are written to provide insight into the discussed event, but with a human touch. The reader will be transported back to another time, looking at the past through the eyes of those who experienced the events.

If you enjoy reading positive, uplifting, and pleasant stories about days gone by, this book is perfect for you. These Narratives are from the 1950s, 1960s, 1970s, 1980s, and 1990s, so you can focus solely on your favorite decade or read them all to reflect on past decades and learn along the way too. Being reminded of long-forgotten events, fads, and more through the eyes of others who experienced them is a great way to keep your memory sharp.

Welcome to the 50s

1. Til Death Do Us Part

The dark-haired woman stood at the end of the bed, smiling at the white silk dress with its bouffant skirt. Her rose point lace veil, handed down by her grandmother, lay across the bed, the tiara adorned with orange blossoms and lace. It was Newport, Rhode Island, on September 12, 1953, and the young woman was about to marry the man she loved in front of 800 guests.

"Are you ready to put your dress on," her sister, Lee, acting as her matron of honor, asked? The young woman nodded, and the bridal party began to help her into the stunning dress. Everyone in the bridal party giggled as they prepared for the big day, the sound drifting through the windows of waves crashing on the beach. After fastening the dress, Lee stood back and looked at her sister.

"You look so beautiful!" she exclaimed as she hugged the dark-haired girl. Nina, the maid of honor and stepsister of the bride, wiped tears from her eyes as Lee placed the tiara on their sister's head. The girl's boarding school roommate, Nancy, picked up the bouquet to hand to her friend as they left the room for the wedding ceremony.

The bride's choker of pearls and the diamond bracelet on her wrist sparkled. The bracelet was a gift from her groom. Hugh, the bride's stepfather, took her arm as they entered the room where the wedding ceremony would occur. The bride smiled shyly as she saw her groom standing tall at the altar, his brother, Bobby, at his side, along with the other groomsmen. His smile was broad, and he would eventually become famous and recognized worldwide, but today it was only for her as she walked toward him down the aisle.

Archbishop Cushing performed the ceremony as the bride and groom stood before their guests. The beautiful bride listened attentively as Luigi Bena sang "Ave Maria" before reciting her vows. Archbishop Cushing announced that the groom could "kiss his bride," Jack did so as the guests applauded. The couple turned to face them as the archbishop made the announcement.

"I present to you, Mr. and Mrs. John Fitzgerald Kennedy."

The couple then headed to their reception on the terrace of the 300-acre estate, celebrating their wedding with 1,200 guests and dancing to the Meyer Davis orchestra in preparation for what should have been a long and happy life together.

The marriage of Jacqueline Bouvier to Senator John F. Kennedy made the national news.

2. Let the Music Take Control

Patty wandered over to the transistor radio on her dresser and turned the knob. It was 1952, and she had just heard about a new disc jockey on Cleveland's WJW Radio. She quickly tuned to the station and heard Alan Freed talking during his Moondog Show.

"Rock 'n roll is really swing with a modern name," she heard the disc jockey say. "It began on the levees and plantations, took in folk songs, and features blues and rhythm. It's the rhythm that gets to the kids. After all those years of crooners, they're starved of music they can dance to."

Patty's eyes grew big as she heard the words. The disc jockey then played that sounded like nothing Patty had ever heard before, a song called "Rock the Joint" by Bill Haley and the Saddlemen. Patty knew the disc jockey was fitting that this music made her want to get up and dance. She began to spin around the room to the music, her skirt swirling around her. The next song began to play, and it made her giggle. "Sixty Minute Man" by the Dominoes was almost risqué, and Patty was excited to talk with her friends about the new music she'd heard.

"Hey, look, if they took it all away tomorrow, we'd be even," said the disc jockey. "No, we wouldn't. We'd be way ahead." Nancy's eyes grew as large as Patty's had listening to the man talk about "rock and roll."

Patty's smile grew, and she looked excited; Patty looked surprised, and she smiled as she realized what the man on the radio was saying. This music was new and exciting.

"What on Earth are you listening to," Nancy's mother said, opening the door. Her face looked shocked at the different sounds coming from the radio.

Patty laughed and explained that this was something called rock and roll.

"This is not appropriate for young ladies," her mother said, appalled at some of the lyrics pouring from the radio. "You need to change that back to a more appropriate station. I don't know who told you this was acceptable, but it is not in this house."

As she left, her mother slammed the door, and Patty rolled her eyes. She knew this music was here to stay.

In 1952, Chicago DJ Alan Freed popularized the term "rock and roll" to describe a new genre of music that combined rhythm and blues with gospel, country, and jazz.

3. A Princess for a Princess

"Daddy! We have to go see this movie!" Mary said, pointing at the poster hanging by the theater as she and her father walked by. The poster showed a pair of mice dancing over the words "Walt Disney's Cinderella." Below that was a girl in a beautiful blue dress dancing with what looked like a prince.

Mary and her father picked up the few items they needed at the hardware store before heading home. Mary ran through the back door, her small patent leather shoes tapping on the linoleum.

"Mommy! Daddy says we can go see a new movie we saw a picture of today!" Mary cried, running up and tugging on her mother's skirt.

Her mother asked Mary to sit at the table to eat lunch as she finished feeding the baby. She wiped his mouth and hands before lifting him from the highchair and slipping him into his walker, where he hurried across the floor. Mary continued to chatter about the beautiful girl in the poster. Mary's mother walked over to the phone in the kitchen and picked it up, dialing a number she knew by heart.

"Hey, Mom? Any chance you can come sit with Johnny for a few hours this afternoon? Mary wants to go see a new movie at the theater, and we thought it would be a nice afternoon out." She nodded and then grinned. "Okay, if you can be over around 3, we can do the late matinee. Thanks, Mom!"

Mary's mother turned toward her daughter.

"Looks like Johnny will be spending time with Grandma while we go see this movie about a girl in a beautiful blue dress," Mary's mother said.

That afternoon, Mary, her father, and her mother loaded into the car to drive to the theater, waving at Grandma and holding Johnny at the door. They got to the theater, and Mary's father paid for their tickets before they headed inside.

The movie began, and Mary sat enthralled as she watched the story unfold. Her eyes welled with tears as she watched Cinderella's stepsisters and stepmother treat her poorly. When the prince slipped the glass slipper on Cinderella's foot, Mary clapped; she was so happy.

On the ride home, Mary sang "Bibbidi-Bobbidi-Boo" in the backseat as her parents smiled, knowing they had just given their princess an afternoon she would never forget.

Walt Disney's Cinderella opened in 1950, and even today, is one of his most critically acclaimed works.

4. A Boy and His Dog

Tommy plopped into his father's recliner, deciding to pretend at least he was a grown-up. He flicked the paper open as he had seen his father do daily. Tommy skipped the boring news articles, quickly arriving at the comics.

"What is this?" he said, noticing a comic he had never seen before. "There is a comic with a dog!" From that day forward, Tommy began to grab the funny pages from his father's newspaper to see what fun Charlie Brown, Lucy, Linus, and Snoopy were getting into.

"Mom, I think we should get a beagle like Snoopy."

"You know that dogs are a lot of work, right?" she asked, drying her hands on her apron. "You will need to take it for walks, feed it, give it baths."

"I promise if we get a dog, I will do it," Tommy said. "But it has to be a beagle. I want a dog like Snoopy!"

That night at dinner, Tommy made his move.

"Dad, I have a question," said Tommy. "If I promise to feed it and walk it and bathe it, can I get a beagle like Snoopy?"

Tommy's father raised an eyebrow as he looked at Tommy's mother.

"I think I may have been ambushed," he said, grinning. "I was wondering why we were having pot roast, which you both know is my favorite, on a weekday evening."

"Hank, I actually think it would be good for Tommy," his mother said. "It would teach him responsibility and would give him a companion."

"If you are willing to take care of a dog, we will head down to the pet store on Saturday and find you that beagle," he said. "But no excuses. The dog will be your responsibility."

"I promise!" he said, reaching over and shaking his father's hand as confirmation.

After breakfast on Saturday, Tommy, his father, and his mother loaded into the car and drove to the pet store. In one cage was a small, black and white beagle puppy who jumped up on the cage when Tommy came close.

“Look! He wants to be my dog!” Tommy said, reaching down to scratch the puppy’s ears.

They left the store with Tommy carrying his new friend.

The “Peanuts” comic strip premiered in newspapers in 1950, the brainchild of Charles Schulz, who patterned Snoopy loosely on his childhood dog, Spike.

5. What Was That?

Ken stood on the porch of his Washington, D.C. home, smoking a cigarette before he turned in for the night. Ken worked on a report at his study desk for several hours. Once he finished, he decided to smoke outside on the porch to take in the warm night air.

It was July 19, 1952, around 11:30 PM, and Ken was sitting on the steps looking at the bright stars. Suddenly, something appeared in the sky, making him look longer. The object looked like an orange ball of fire with a tail traveling at a high rate of speed. Soon after, the orange ball seemed to vanish, and several smaller, white objects appeared. The more minor things did not have a tail but seemed moving in a formation.

“I must really be overworked,” Ken thought to himself as he snuffed out the cigarette and headed inside the house to bed.

The next day, Ken was stunned to see headlines in the paper that read “Saucers Swarm Over Capital.” According to the documents, air traffic controllers and several pilots had seen the same things in the sky that he saw. Ken was not convinced weather conditions caused what he saw.

About a week later, Ken was sitting on a flight returning from a short business trip at the National Airport. He glanced out the window and saw the same white lights he had seen while sitting on his front porch. He pointed them out to a stewardess who explained that the pilot had also seen them and that the objects had been radioed to the tower. Ken was convinced that he had seen alien spacecraft.

“I am telling you, Judith, what I saw was not a shooting star,” he told his wife a few days later. “It did not have the streaks or tails like a shooting star would have. It was balls of light that all moved together. It was almost like when they saw the plane; they disappeared; it was so fast.”

“It says right there it was weather,” Judith said, pointing at the paper.

“I know what I saw,” he insisted, shaking his head.
On July 29, a press conference was held regarding the UFO sightings in Washington. Ken watched raptly to hear what he may have seen, only to be disappointed when a general claimed the objects were stars or meteors.

From July 12 to 29, 1952, several unidentified flying objects (UFOs) were seen over Washington D.C., but the government claimed *they were either weather phenomenon or meteors.*

6. Climb Every Mountain

Edmund stood on the icy face of the mountain, knowing that dozens of expeditions like his had failed before. His sherpa, Tenzing, walked over to him, ice crunching under his feet.

“We should be heading off soon, sir,” Tenzing said, standing beside the tall, commanding gentleman.

Edmund smiled, still taking in the view and thinking back on what led him to these accomplishments. This was his most challenging climb yet, and two climbers had failed to reach the summit just the day before.

“At least the snow and wind seem to have stopped,” Edmund said as they stood in the small camp, they built almost 30,000 feet above the Earth. The cold was almost unbearable that morning, his boots were frozen to the ground, and he had to chip the ice before putting them on.

The two men packed up the camp and strapped on their gear. They headed upward until they reached a 40-foot rock face.

“There is a crack between the rock and the snow to the east,” Edmund said. “I believe we can crawl inside and work our way to the top.”

Edmund slipped into the crevice, chopping steps into the ice with Tenzing behind him for hours. He wondered if he would ever see the summit when suddenly, the ridge head disappeared, and a rounded snow dome appeared. Edmund dug into the ice several times and stepped out of the aperture.

On May 28, 1953, Edmund Hillary was the first to stand at the highest point on Earth, with Tenzing Norgay just a few steps behind him. The two men spent just 15 minutes on Mount Everest, with Tenzing leaving chocolates as an offering. Edmund left a cross given to him by fellow climber John Hunt. The descent to base camp was hampered by snow, but the two men knew they had conquered the mountain many thought could never be defeated.

Sir Edmund Hillary and Tenzing Norgay were the first to stand atop Mount Everest, the tallest mountain on Earth.

7. Creating a Best Friend

Jim sat at the table, contemplating the myriad of items before him. He had just signed a contract for a new show called *Sam and Friends* which would feature puppets, something Jim had developed an interest in while attending college. His vision for this new show was to break the mold and showcase puppets unlike anything ever seen before.

"Puppets carved from wood just don't appear alive," Jim told his girlfriend, Jane. "I want these to have life, to be able to express emotions. I just need to figure out how to make that happen."

On the table was an old green coat that belonged to his mother and ping pong balls. Suddenly, Jim had an idea. He began to cut up the skin into the shape of a frog. He found some foam rubber in a closet and trimmed it into the shape of the coat material. Jim sewed everything together, cut a ping pong ball in half, and attached them to the head of his new puppet. He also attached rods to his puppet's arms instead of the string used by most puppeteers.

"Instead of the regular camera angles, let's try putting live feed monitors on the floor," Jim said. "That way, we can see the puppets the same way the audience does."

Sam and Friends premiered in 1955 and featured Sam, a bald man who escaped everyday life with abstract friends. His friends, all created by Jim, included Yorick, Harry the Hipster, Professor Madcliffe, and Chicken Liver. Soon after the premiere, the show featured a lizard frog, the puppet created from Jim's mother's coat, and a ping pong ball.

"I am Kermit," the puppet said, voiced by Jim himself.

As the show progressed, Kermit became an instant celebrity with viewers. Jim could contort the puppet's face so that it appeared his creation had actual feelings and emotions. There is no question that when Jim cut up his mother's old coat and put ping pong balls on it for eyes, he created a star.

Kermit the Frog was introduced on Sam and Friends in 1955, originally looking more like a lizard. In fact, he was not called a frog until 1969.

8. The Road Trip

"Children, wake up," Betty and Gary heard their mother say. Both of them sat up and looked out the car window. It was light now, not pitch dark like when they loaded into the car in the early morning hours.

They were in the parking lot of a diner that looked almost like a train car. A sign in front of the restaurant said, “Route 66.” The four of them headed inside.

“How long will it take to get to California?” Gary asked as he ate his waffles with strawberries and whipped cream.

“About three days,” his father said. “We will spend the night tonight and tomorrow night at hotels. Mother has packed a bunch of good food, so we shouldn’t need to stop to eat again until breakfast tomorrow.”

After they ate, they began their journey again, the children playing “I Spy” and coloring in the books that their mother brought to keep them occupied. They laughed at some of the funny attractions they saw along the way, and their eyes grew wide at the warnings about “Dead Man’s Curve.” They stopped at a small picnic area where they ate a lunch of bologna sandwiches.

Soon, Father saw a sign for a motel in a town called Elk City. Father went into the office and came back with a key. They pulled the car in front of a room with the same number on the door that was on the key.

The room had two double beds and a dresser with a television sitting on it. There was a closet and a door that led to a small bathroom. A table with two chairs was seated by the window, and Father placed the ice chest next to it before returning to the car and bringing in a giant suitcase.

Mother fixed each of them a plate of chicken and salad. She handed each child a glass from the tray on the dresser and told them to get water from the bathroom to drink. She gave them a homemade chocolate chip cookie when they finished their meals.

Father was looking at a paper with many squiggly lines on it. Betty asked what he was doing.

“This is a map of where we are going,” Father said. “We are right here. Tomorrow, we want to be at least this far.” Betty pretended to understand what all the lines meant, but the day's excitement was too much, and her eyes grew heavy. Gary was already asleep next to Father.

Their adventure had just begun.

During the 1950s, Route 66 became a main highway for vacationers, and many families traveled the road on their way to Los Angeles.

9. Shake Your Hips

“Joyce! You have got to see this thing I just bought!” Martha said, coming down the steps with a massive plastic ring.

Joyce sat her teacup on the saucer as Martha handed the ring to her, her eyes wide.

“What does this thing do?” she asked.

“It’s called a Hula Hoop!” Martha said. She took the ring from Joyce and stepped inside it. “You are supposed to put it around your waist and shake your hips to make it spin around.”

“How on Earth can that work?” Joyce asked. Martha laughed and told her to watch.

Martha held the ring with one hand close to her body and began to spin it; she then moved her hips quickly in a circle as the hoop started to turn around in time with her motions. It fell within a few seconds, but Joyce was excited.

“That looks so neat! Let me try!” Joyce said, and Martha handed her the hoop.

Martha and Joyce had succumbed to the hula hoop craze. It was not long before Joyce purchased her hula hoop, and the two women began competing to see who could keep the circle spinning longer. Although the toy was marketed to children, adults also began to use the spinning hoops.

“I saw them using the hula hoop on the *Steve Allen Show*,” Martha told Joyce one day over coffee. “I think there should be some kind of official competition for these things.” It was not long before hula hoop competitions began appearing around their area and across the country. Martha and Joyce even competed in a local contest, with Martha edging Joyce out by just a few seconds.

The Hula Hoop was released by Wham-O in 1958, selling for $1.98 each, and the toy became an instant sensation.

10. Living in a Barbie World

The doll looked like no other doll Gloria had ever seen, and as soon as she saw an advertisement for it during her favorite show, *The Mickey Mouse Club*, she knew she had to have one. Even the box she came in was fashionable, with photos of beautiful outfits that could be purchased for the doll.

Barbie became Gloria's favorite toy, and she loved it when her mother would surprise her with new clothes for the doll. Mother made most of the clothes herself but sometimes splurged on sets of shoes and purses so that Gloria's Barbie was one of the best dressed among her friends. Gloria began to immerse herself in Barbie's world, collecting everything she could.
With Barbie, Gloria could pretend she could have everything and anything she wanted. Barbie was the epitome of sophistication. Her fashion booklet detailed how vital hygiene and homemaking were for women, but Barbie herself seemed above these things.

Her room became a haven for Gloria as she developed elaborate stories involving Barbie. Her mother splurged and purchased the official wedding gown for the doll, and Gloria used a "Bob" doll similar to Barbie to act as the doll's husband.

In Gloria's fantasy world, Barbie became the person Gloria wanted to be. She was a doctor, a lawyer, a teacher, and a mother as Gloria made up stories about babies for Barbie and Bob. As she grew older, Barbie was set aside, and Gloria began to pursue her goals and dreams, many rooted in her playacting with Barbie.

Her obsession with a doll led Gloria to finish as valedictorian of her high school class and become the first woman in her family to attend college. Just as she'd used her imagination to create a variety of careers and adventures for Barbie in her small bedroom, Gloria could achieve goals that she may not have even considered had it not been for the small plastic doll.

Barbie was released by Mattel in 1959, the creation of Ruth Handler, and named for her daughter.

11. The Fear Can Subside

The two women watched their children play in the park, grateful they could again do so. Until a few weeks ago, mothers kept their children home from playgrounds and even school to prevent them from contracting polio, a dangerous virus that was paralyzing some children and killing others. Still, others needed to be in iron lungs which allowed them to breathe.

"I have missed bringing Wayne out to the playground," one mother said. The other agreed, mentioning that her older son had not been able to play baseball for months, and he was driving her crazy.

All summer, fears about polio spreading had been disrupting everyone's lives across the country. Signs were erected outside of towns warning visitors that there was an outbreak. This led many travelers to ride in stifling hot cars rather than risk breathing "polio air."

Then, it was announced that a man named Jonas Salk had discovered a vaccine to stop the spread of polio. As soon as it was available, people lined up to get the shot not only to protect their children but to protect themselves as well.

"As soon as they announced it was available, we were in line," Wayne's mother said. "I did not want our kids to end up confined to an iron lung or have to walk with crutches and canes for the rest of their life."

Joe's mother agreed.

“The daughter of a cousin had polio, and she will never walk again,” the woman said, tears forming in her eyes.

Thanks to Dr Jonas Salk and his discovery, the number of polio cases fell to less than 100 by 1960. Dr. Jonas Salk discovered the polio vaccine in 1953, and it was first tested on school children in 1954. The vaccine brought an end to the fear many felt regarding the polio virus.

12. Dinner in Front of the Television

Joan walked down the grocery store's aisles, her list in her hand. Her pumps clicked on the tile floor, her skirt swishing around her legs as she pulled items from the shelf, tossed them in the cart, and crossed them off the list.

“After working all day, I am just too tired to cook,” she thought. “I sure wish there was a quick meal other than sandwiches.”

Joan turned the corner into the frozen food aisle and reached for a box of vegetables. Out of the corner of her eye, she saw an item she had never seen before. A flat box with the Swanson brand name and a photo of sliced turkey, sweet potatoes, gravy, stuffing, and peas. The words “TV Dinner” were emblazoned in one corner, and the box looked like a television set.

“Well, what is this?” Joan wondered, opening the freezer door and pulling out the package. The price was less than one dollar, so Joan grabbed two of them, one for herself and one for her husband, George.

After unloading the groceries when she got home, Joan looked at the directions on the box. She set the oven temperature as directed and pulled the tray with the food out of the box. It looked appetizing, and Joan was incredibly excited that the metal tray could simply be tossed in the trash after dinner, leaving only the utensils they used to eat for her to wash. The oven reached the set temperature, and she slid the two trays inside, setting the timer for 25 minutes.

“We'll make this an adventure,” Joan thought. She entered the living room and opened two TV trays they used occasionally.

George came in and dropped his briefcase on the table by the front door before wandering into the kitchen to kiss Joan. His eyebrows rose as he saw what she pulled from the oven.

“What is this?” he asked. Joan set the metal trays on the TV tables and walked over to turn on the television, where Douglas Edwards appeared, reading the evening news.

“This is a TV Dinner; they are brand new,” Joan said, taking her seat and gesturing for George to take his. George looked skeptical as he sat down in his chair. He scooped up some of the potatoes and took a bite.

“This is delicious!” he told Joan enjoying one of the first TV dinners on the market.

Swanson was the first to mass market TV dinners which became a staple in the homes of many people in the 1950s.

13. Going to School

James and Margaret were ecstatic when they heard the news. The Supreme Court had ruled that their son, Harry, would no longer be required to attend a school just for black children. The decision the news was calling Brown v. Board of Education had been decided, and schools would now have to admit both black and white students.

Their elation was short-lived, however, when the public school system shut down in their area of Virginia, and a private white-only school opened up instead.

"Our son needs to continue his education," James said to Margaret one evening as they ate dinner. James owned his own business, a small general store in their town, while Margaret cleaned the homes of the rich. They held their home and were highly regarded in the community. James completed high school at the local black-only facility, while Margaret dropped out in the ninth grade. Both wanted a better life for their young son.

A few days later, after attending church, Harriet, a teacher at the black high school, came up to James and Margaret.

"I want to open a community center where I can offer classes to students," Harriet said. "It won't be the same as a real school, but at least our children will get some semblance of education until this all winds through the court system."

Less than a week later, Harry sat in a pew at the church with Harriet at the altar, teaching him and other black children multiplication tables, spelling, and more. Eventually, Harry was able to take a college placement test and qualified to attend a local black college. This small community school, created after the Supreme Court ruled that schools should be desegregated, allowed Harry to become the first person in his family to attend and graduate from college.

Harry earned a law degree and was instrumental in helping schools in his area desegregate after the Supreme Court officially required all districts to do so.

Although Brown v. Education required schools in the United States to desegregate, the language was vague and allowed areas of the country to delay implementation, and some communities actually shut down schools to avoid complying.

14. Walt's Dream

Sitting on a park bench in Griffith Park, Walt watched his children riding the carousel. Although Walt had already become famous because of the cartoons he created, he wanted to expand his creativity and build a park where families could be together. He was even receiving letters from fans who wanted to tour the studios, but Walt knew that the actual animation studio was not as fascinating as people believed.

"I'm going to create an amusement park that is clean, friendly, and geared toward families," Walt told his wife that evening. Lillian smiled at him.

“If anyone can build a park that meets all those requirements, dear, it is you,” Lillian said to her husband after being by his side when everyone else told him his dreams would never come true.

An idea began forming in Walt’s head, so he sat down and wrote a memo to a production designer, telling Dick that he wanted to create a family-friendly theme park, unlike those that existed currently. The original plan was for a boat ride, and some themed areas, but the vision overgrew. Walt purchased land for the park, and construction began.

After a year of construction, the park opened on July 17, 1955, with 18 rides and attractions, but Walt was stunned when the first day of his new park was a disaster. It was scorching that day and many people trying to enter the park had forged tickets. Some were even jumping fences to get in. The asphalt had not been allowed to set, and the female guests’ high heels were sinking into the pavement. A plumber’s strike forced Walt to decide between having operational bathrooms or water fountains. The list of problems on that first day was endless. But Walt was not deterred by the difficulties.

“To all who come to this happy place: Welcome! Disneyland is your land. Here age relives fond memories of the past, and here youth may savor the challenge and promise of the future. Disneyland is dedicated to the ideals, the drama, and the hard facts that have created America, with the hope that it will be a source of joy and inspiration to all the world.”

What began as Walt’s Folly has since become one of the happiest places on Earth, Disneyland.

Disneyland was originally named the Mickey Mouse Park and then Disneylandia until Walt Disney settled on the official name.

15. There She Is, Miss America

Evelyn felt like she was far from her hometown of Ephrata, Pennsylvania. Despite living so close, she had never been to Atlantic City before nor had she ever seen the ocean.

“This hotel is so beautiful!” Evelyn told her mother as they walked through the lobby; her father was talking to the bellhop who was getting their luggage. Evelyn carried the garment bag protecting her evening gown, as she did not want it to get wrinkled. There was a table to the left of the lobby with a sign that read “Miss America,” so Evelyn walked over.

“Welcome!” a cheerful woman said. She took Evelyn’s name, checking it off a list before her. She handed Evelyn a packet of information and a hotel room key. Evelyn’s mother and father joined her after checking into their room since Evelyn would have to room with another contestant.

The weekend was a whirlwind of activity, and Evelyn loved every second. Finally, the big night arrived, and Evelyn strolled across the stage first in a snug bathing suit, then in the evening gown she had insisted on hand-carrying to protect it when they arrived. Finally, she performed in front of the audience and judges. She walked off the stage, knowing she had done her best.

The girls were jittery and nervous as the judges made their decision. It did not help that millions were watching them as this pageant was being televised for the first time. They listened as the Top 10 finalists were announced, and Evelyn was shocked to hear her name called. The girls held hands as Susanne from Mississippi was announced as the fourth runner-up and then Virginia from

Alabama. Anne from Virginia was advertised as the second runner-up, leaving Evelyn and Joan from New York trembling on the stage as hundreds watched in the audience and millions on television.

"Miss America 1954 is Miss Pennsylvania!" the announcer said as the audience applauded. Evelyn initially stood rooted to the spot as Joan hugged her. The tears began to fall as Miss America 1953, Neva placed the crown on her head, and Evelyn was handed a bouquet of roses. The music started to play, and Evelyn walked across the stage, knowing her life had just changed forever.

The Miss America pageant was first televised on ABC in 1954.

16. The Dream House

The young man walked into the formal front room of the large house and looked around in awe. Sitting in one corner was a large harp, and the furnishings were beautiful.

"The daughter of the current owner played with the orchestra," the real estate broker told the young man. "I imagine they will be taking that with them."

As they walked through the formal dining room, the younger man stopped to admire the black marble floor.

"So how did this place get its name," the young man asked slowly with the typical pacing of a distinct Southern drawl, his voice low.

"It was named after the niece of the original owner when it was built in 1939," the real estate broker said. "Will you be living here alone?"

"No, I plan to live here with my family, my mother, and father will be moving in with me," the young man said. "What else can you tell me about this house?"

"It was built by Dr Thomas D. Moore on land gifted to them by his wife's parents," the real estate agent said. "The house was designed by Furbringer and Ehrman and built for just over $41,000. When they divorced, Mrs Moore allowed a church to use the home until they built the one on adjacent land, but they left some of the furnishings here."

The young man smiled, taking in the stunning features of the home. He loved the quietness of the location and the breathtaking beauty of the house. Each of the 28 rooms was a marvel of beauty to him after growing up poor. He had been living on Audubon Drive in a lovely house not far from the Dixon Gallery and Gardens but wanted something more private. Just 22 years old, the young man had become extremely famous over the past year, and he simply wanted a place where he could relax with his family and friends away from the public eye.

"I love this place," he told the real estate agent, Virginia Grant after they completed the mansion tour, including the four-car garage. "Let me go home and talk to my family."

Just a few days later, Elvis Presley purchased Graceland and created a home that was a bit lavish, a bit flashy, but was the place he considered home. It was where he brought his new bride Priscilla a few years later and then his beloved daughter, Lisa Marie.

Elvis purchased Graceland in March 1957 for $102,500, adding the now iconic music note gates and a swimming pool after he moved into the mansion.

17. Let's Go Shopping

"We have to go see what it's like!" Susie said on the telephone when speaking with her friend Gina. The Southdale Center had just opened up in nearby Edina. Susie's husband, Frank, was away on a business trip and left her money to buy new clothing. Gina was a new mother, always looking for new items for the baby.

"We could just go downtown and visit JCPenney or W.T. Grant," Gina said, knowing that Susie would never agree to shop in the stores they usually went to now that this fancy new shopping option had opened just a few miles away.

"Not a chance! What if it rains? We'd need umbrellas and raincoats. This is indoors, Gina! We can park the car and just wander around for hours without worrying about the weather!" Gina laughed, and the two women agreed to meet at Susie's house on Saturday morning.

Sure enough, when Gina arrived at Susie's house, it was drizzling rain predicted to turn to snow later that afternoon. Susie hopped into Gina's car, and they headed to the new mall. It was a huge building, and the parking lot was already filling up when the women arrived. They pulled the stroller out of the back of the station wagon and strapped baby Lisa into the stroller, walking quickly to avoid getting too wet.

Inside, the mall was bustling with activity. The women wandered through Dayton's and then visited some of the smaller stores before heading into Donaldson's, where Gina found cute outfits for Lisa. They then strolled to Woolworth's, where they enjoyed lunch at the counter, sharing a milkshake for dessert. The two women then walked around the garden court and stopped to look at the Sidewalk Café, an outdoor-style restaurant entirely indoors.

Once they were finished shopping, the women pushed the stroller back to the car amid light snow, loading the baby in the backseat and heading home. When they arrived at Susie's, she looked at Gina and grinned.

"I think we have just found our new favorite shopping location," Susie said, leaning over and kissing Gina on the cheek before heading back inside the house.

The first indoor shopping mall opened in Edina, Minnesota, on October 8, 1956.

18. A Princess Becomes Queen

Shirley fought back tears as she sat in the back of Westminster Abbey. She could not believe she was about to see history being made. When she was young, her mother had been fascinated by Queen Victoria, an interest she passed along to her young daughter. As a result, Shirley followed the monarchy closely through all of Queen Victoria's successors. She wept when King Edward VII, affectionately known as Bertie, died suddenly, placing his younger brother, George, on the throne.

When George V was coronated, Shirley stood outside the Abbey with thousands of others, too young to get inside. When King George died, she again wept and stood outside Westminster Hall as the king lay in state. She, along with the rest of England, was shocked when Edward, King George's son, stepped down from the throne to marry his beloved Wallis Simpson, thrusting his younger brother onto the throne.

Shirley became enamored with the young princesses in the castle. Princess Elizabeth and her younger sister, Princess Margaret, were living the fairy tale that all young girls dream of, wandering the halls of Buckingham Palace as the daughters of the new king. Married now with two young girls, Shirley was considered royalty herself, as her husband was related to the Windsor family. She was at home when she learned of the death of King George, and she wept as she thought of the two young girls who were now fatherless.

Several days later, Shirley was thrilled when she and her husband received word they were invited to the coronation of the young queen. As Shirley sat in the back row, she thought about the flight from Kenya Elizabeth had taken after learning of her father's death. Her heart broke for her on that day, but today was a joyous occasion. She smiled as the soon-to-be Queen Elizabeth walked to the front of the Abbey and stood before the Archbishop of Canterbury. Her heart swelled with pride as she recalled the words of young Elizabeth that played on the radio the night before.

"Throughout all my life and with all my heart, I shall strive to be worthy of your trust."

Shirley smiled widely as she sat in her seat, her husband next to her, as she heard her new monarch utter the words she had been waiting to hear.

"I swear to maintain and preserve inviolably the settlement of the Church of England, and the doctrine worship, discipline and government thereof, as the law established in England," Elizabeth recited.

After the ceremony, Shirley's eyes filled with tears as she watched Queen Elizabeth's new husband pay homage to her. She took in the stunning circlet of diamonds the new queen wore as St. Edward's Crown was placed on her head, her hands gripping a bouquet of orchids, lilies-of-the-valley, stephanotis, and carnations.

Shirley joined the rest of the world in rejoicing as they watched the coronation of Queen Elizabeth II.

Princess Elizabeth took the throne when her father, Prince George VI, died, and her coronation was held June 2, 1953.

19. The Beginning

Janie handed the group at the small table their drinks, watching as the tall thin man on stage played his guitar and sang. As a waitress at The Cavern Club, she was familiar with the young man as he had been playing there almost every weekend since she could remember. He finished his song and told the audience he was taking a break.

"That was great, John," Janie said, handing him a pint. "You get better and better every week."

John took a sip and grinned at the young waitress.

"I have this weird gig in a few days, though," John said. "A friend wants us to play at a church thing. Ivy said it was going to be a lot of fun. Why don't you join us?" Janie told John she would be off that evening, so she would be able to go.

The night of the gathering, John and his band, the Quarryman, played a doo-wop song called "Come Go With Me," but with lyrics John improvised. A young man named Paul walked up to introduce himself. As they waited to retake the stage, Paul asked for a go at John's guitar. The young man returned the instrument and turned it upside down so he could play left-handed. He then played a version of "Twenty Flight Back," a song by Eddie Cochran.

John, only 15 himself, was impressed with the spunky 16-year-old Paul. John noticed a slight resemblance to the American rocker Elvis, but Paul had significantly more talent, able to play the guitar and the piano. Janie knew she was watching history in the making as the two teens played several songs together.

Just a few weeks later, John asked Paul to become a member of the Quarrymen. Janie watched as they often played the Canyon but was soon following them to The Casbah Coffee Club and the Jacaranda Club to listen to the original songs written by John and Paul. Janie knew it would not be long before John and Paul became household names.

Janie was correct as the two teens who met that day, performing what was known as skiffle music at St. Peter's Church, would become one of the most prolific song-writing duos of all time.

John Lennon met Paul McCartney at a church hall concert when the two were just young teens.

20. Because of Misty

Audrey stood at the door of the stable, looking down the row of horse stalls. She drew deep breath, smelling the fresh hay and horses inside. She strolled down the center, smiling at the magnificent animals inside each stall.

"Good morning, Sea Star, hello, Stormy," she said as the horses seemed to nod back at her. She reached the end stall to find Misty, her regal head bouncing as Audrey called her. She patted her nose and handed her the apple tucked in her other hand.

Audrey had loved horses since she was a young girl, growing up on the Eastern Shore of Maryland. There was no question where her love of horses came from as it developed as soon as she read *Misty of Chincoteague*. The story of the spunky pony who grew up on the Beebe Ranch in Chincoteague, Virginia, immediately wormed its way into Audrey's heart. She read the first book when she was only eight years old and read every other book in the series afterwards. She had read all of them multiple times.

While attending high school, Audrey knew she wanted to work with horses and decided to become a veterinarian. While at college, she could work on a horse farm, and when the owner was ready to retire, he worked out a deal with Audrey to let her purchase the farm.

Her veterinary practice grew, and Audrey continued to add horses to her stables. Each horse was named after a horse in the Misty series. Then, one day, she heard on the news that Misty was returning to Chincoteague to live out her years on the Beebe ranch.

Audrey knew she had to see the pony who created her love of horses.

Audrey arrived on the island after crossing the small drawbridge. She guided her car to the Beebe Ranch, where she purchased a ticket for admission to visit the horse that meant so much to her. Even as an adult, Audrey was in awe of the famous horse before her.

Misty stood, her head high, as people watched her. The markings on her side resembling a United States map were still prominent. Audrey was surprised to see how small Misty actually was since, in her mind, the horse stood very tall. The fact was that Chincoteague ponies were more miniature than the average horse, something that Audrey did not know until she saw Misty for herself.

As soon as she could get close, she spoke directly to Misty, letting her know that her namesake lived with her not far north of the island. Audrey was able to pat Misty's nose, and she felt that the horse responded to her.

Audrey left the island with tears streaming down her cheeks, knowing that the small horse in the corral on the Beebe Ranch had changed her life forever.

Misty of Chincoteague was a book published by Marguerite Henry which gained popularity in the 1950s.

Welcome to the 60s

1. A Man on the Moon

Frank called to his children in the yard playing on a sunny Sunday afternoon. When they ran inside, they were surprised to see the television on since it was Sunday, and their father insisted the television remain off during the day.

"Children, this is one of the most important things you will ever watch," Frank said. "Sit down in front of the television and just watch what happens."

Sandy, Grace, and Frankie plopped on the floor in front of the television, unsure of what was so crucial that Father had the television that afternoon. They heard what sounded like people talking underwater and on the screen, they saw a strange-looking spacecraft perched on what appeared to be rocks and dirt.

"Back many years ago, President Kennedy issued a challenge to the space agency to land on the moon," Frank explained. "We have been working on making that happen, especially since President Kennedy died without ever seeing it happen. Frank, an engineer for one of the space agency contractors, was particularly thrilled to watch this dream become a reality.

"The Eagle has landed," they all heard through the television speakers. They heard more chattering from what must have been the people in the spacecraft and those still on Earth waiting for the men to exit the craft. A door opened, and a man in a spacesuit stepped out the door.

"I'm going to step off the LM now," they heard the man say, his voice sounding strange through his helmet. "That's one small step for man, one giant leap for mankind." Frank's face broke into a huge smile as he saw Neil Armstrong take the first steps on the moon.

"The surface is fine and powdery," they heard the man say. "I can — I can pick it up loosely with my toe. It does adhere in fine layers like powdered charcoal to the sole and sides of my boots. I only go in a small fraction of an inch. Maybe an eighth of an inch, but I can see the footprints of my boots and the treads in the fine sandy particles."

The children were shocked and amazed as a second man stepped out of the spaceship and walked out on the moon's surface. Frank knew that the world would never be the same after this accomplishment.

Neil Armstrong and Buzz Aldrin were the first men to walk on the surface of the moon on July 16, 1969.

2. The French Chef

Judy sat in her small apartment, using her spoon to stir the bowl of soup she had heated up from a can for her dinner, realizing her dream of becoming an actress was slowly dimming. Sighing, she decided to turn on the television as a distraction.

"Learn how to cook," a woman with a very high-pitched voice said. "Try new recipes, learn from your mistakes, be fearless, and above all, have fun." The woman stood in what appeared to be a kitchen, stirring a pot on a stove. Judy leaned forward to pay more attention.

The woman added butter to her cooking, talking as she did. Then, she began to laugh.

“Well, goodness, that was a little more butter than I wanted.” Judy, who had always enjoyed cooking, giggled as well, watching the woman chatter as she added ingredients. Judy glanced at the clock and realized it was time to head to her shift in the restaurant down the street, but now she had a new idea.

That night at work, she chatted with the chef about his experiences in the kitchen. She mentioned watching the cooking show, and he laughed.

“You must have watched *The French Chef* with Julia Child,” he said. “She has grown quite famous, and you could learn a lot from watching her.”

From that point on, Judy made a point to watch Julia learning to debone a whole chicken with just a few knife cuts, how to make fancy dishes like Tarte Tatin, and what spices blended well with various foods. Judy learned how to make crepes and souffles, often heading to the restaurant early for her shift to practice what she had learned with the chef.

One night, Judy arrived for her shift and headed to the kitchen. The chef stopped what he was doing and looked at Judy.

“I have talked to the manager, and we have decided you would make a great sous chef,” he said. “I am not sure how you are learning such intricate cooking techniques so easily, but you are extremely talented.”

From then on, Judy began working in the restaurant kitchen, side-by-side with the chef, which helped increase her skills even more.

She continued to watch Julia and implemented much of what she learned from the woman on television in the restaurant kitchen. Five years later, Judy became the head chef at that restaurant and eventually opened her own, growing her culinary franchise over the years.

Julia Child's show, the French Chef, premiered February 11, 1963, and became an instant success, inspiring many people to enter the culinary field.

3. "I Have a Dream"

Standing in the crowd in front of the Lincoln Memorial, Lionel and his friends were checking out the public. The boys had skipped school to see all the excitement about this man who seemed to have everyone talking, especially in the predominantly black neighborhood where they lived. Suddenly, the crowd began to cheer, and Lionel looked at the large memorial before him.

"Five score years ago, a great American, in whose symbolic shadow we stand today, signed the Emancipation Proclamation," Dr King began. "It came as a joyous daybreak to end the long night of their captivity."

Lionel stopped chatting with his friends and turned his attention to the speech. He had never heard such passion when someone spoke.

"When the architects of our republic wrote the magnificent words of the Constitution and the Declaration of Independence, they were signing a promissory note to which every American was to fall heir," Dr King continued. "This note was a promise that all men — yes, black men as well as white men — would be guaranteed the unalienable rights of life, liberty, and the pursuit of happiness."

Dr King continued, urging those in the crowd to remain steadfast in their fight for civil rights. He explained that gaining justice did not mean he encouraged people to drink from a cup of bitterness and hatred. He urged those listening to fight with dignity and discipline, not stoop to physical violence.

"Let us not wallow in the valley of despair, I say to you today, my friends," Dr King said. "So even though we face the difficulties of today and tomorrow, I still have a dream. It is a dream deeply rooted in the American dream. I dream that one day this nation will rise and live out the true meaning of its creed: We hold these truths to be self-evident, that all men are created equal."

Lionel, his friends, and the rest of the crowd erupted in cheers as Dr King concluded his speech.

When he heard Dr. Martin Luther King, Jr. speak, Lionel's life was never the same. He eventually became a minister.

Dr Martin Luther King, Jr. gave his impassioned "I Have a Dream" speech on August 28, 1963, a speech that became an anthem for people of color throughout the world.

4. The Concert on the Farm

After hitchhiking from Virginia, Luke and Dan arrived in Bethel, New York. While sitting in a small café, they heard about a music festival that was supposed to start in a few days.

“A three-day music festival?” Luke said, shaking his head. “Man, there is no way that is ever going to happen. But, what the heck? Let’s go see what it is all about.”

The men heard tickets could be purchased at a few record stores in town, but most people were going without them. They decided just to risk it and hitchhiked their way to the field.

Once there, Luke and Dan kicked back in the dusty field in front of a stage that looked still under construction. They walked directly into the concert arena without tickets as there was no fencing or ticket booths to block them. It had been raining off and on, and the result was a muddy mess at the concert.

When the music began on Friday, the two men relaxed to the sounds of Richie Havens, even though they had heard it would be the band Sweetwater. However, that band was delayed by traffic. Melanie, Arlo Guthrie, and Joan Baez all took the stage that day as Luke and Dan joined several groups of other people, of other concertgoers, all developing friendships they knew would last a lifetime.

The men slept on their bedrolls in a less muddy spot than others. The next day, they danced to Santana, Canned Heat, the Grateful Dead, and Creedence Clearwater before Janis Joplin took the stage. Sly and the Family Stone, The Who, and Jefferson Airplane continued the performances until 2 PM on Sunday when Joe Cocker took the step. The music continued throughout the night, ending with Jimi Hendrix and his now famous "Star Spangled Banner" rendition.

After the concert ended, Luke found that he loved the area. Dan moved on, hitchhiking back to Virginia, but Luke found a job at a local record store. While working in the store, he met his future wife. The couple remained in Bethel the rest of their lives, always remembering the three-day music festival 1969 that kept Luke in New York.

The Woodstock Music and Art Fair was held August 15 through 18, 1969, attracting more than 400,000 attendees.

5. Can You Tell Me How to Get...

Fran finally got the baby down for a nap and decided that turning on the television to distract her three-year-old was justifiable today. Fran needed to get the ironing done, and Chester had been clinging to her all day for some reason. With Clara asleep, she felt turning on the television might keep Chester occupied while she ironed in the same room.

She flipped to the local PBS station and saw a new children's show that she had not seen. She sat Chester on the floor in front of the set and opened the ironing board. The show began with two boys named David and Donald arriving on a city street. A man who was walking on the sidewalk introduced himself as Gordon. Chester was captivated as in between scenes with the two boys, and the show focused on words that started with "D."

Fran was captivated as she watched unique puppets teach her son about counting and the alphabet. That night, over dinner, she told her husband about this exciting children's show that entertained Chester and kept her giggling.

Over the next few years, Fran allowed her children to watch the show regularly. She found that Chester began recognizing letters much sooner than her friend's children, that were the same age. Clara, who started watching the show with Chester as soon as she was old enough to pay attention, also seemed to be more advanced regarding letters, numbers, and colors.

The children were fascinated with the antics of Big Bird, Oscar the Grouch, Kermit the Frog, Bert, and Ernie. Fran began to enjoy watching the show as much as her children did, realizing that the puppets were teaching them valuable lessons and preparing them for school.

Many years passed, and Fran's children seemed to outgrow the silliness of the characters, but the lessons they learned remained. When Chester graduated from high school, he went to college and earned a degree in education. He told his mother that one of the main reasons he did so was because of the lessons he learned on that child's television show. His sister, Clara, became a social worker after seeing how the show handled the death of a character.

Chester and Clara were just two of millions of children who discovered how to get to Sesame Street and developed a lifelong love of learning because, one busy afternoon, their mother turned on the television as a distraction.

Sesame Street debuted on November 10, 1969, changing children's television programming forever.

6. A Soup Can

Audrey walked down the street, the clothing and other items catching her eye as she passed. She stopped when she reached the Ferus Gallery and saw the painting of a giant soup can. As an artist, Audrey was intrigued by the commercial art displayed in what had always been a fine art gallery. She stepped inside to look around.

Inside the gallery, Audrey was enthralled by the unique paintings she saw. In addition to the iconic soup cans, there were paintings of Coca-Cola bottles and soap pad boxes. The entire show seemed like a pop-art display, something she had never seen. The gallery owner walked out when he saw Audrey's expression.

"Pretty unusual, isn't it?" he said. Audrey nodded her head.

"This is the work of Andy Warhol, an up-and-coming artist," he told her. "I don't know if you have ever heard of 'The Factory,' but it is what he calls his studio. Creative people get together there and make very impactful art. Andy sees artists as designers, not just people with artistic talent."

Audrey looked around her at the various paintings that depicted everyday items.

"This is almost a social commentary," Audrey said. "It depicts how we are all consumers and that consumer-related items can be just as artistic as a painting of a bowl of fruit." Audrey left the gallery with new inspiration for her art.

Returning home to her studio, Audrey pulled out her paints and canvas, using broad brush strokes to develop a painting that depicted her feelings. It was an abstract, but she knew what she created was impactful. Over the next few weeks, Audrey created several similar paintings. She then carried a few pictures to show a local gallery owner who she felt might showcase her work.

"These are outstanding!" the gallery owner told her. "This is so unlike your previous work. It is bold, forceful, and unique." Audrey beamed at his compliments. A showing was planned for the following month.

Her showing was a success, and Audrey sold many of her paintings at the gallery. Her style shifted so that her paintings were more along the bold, bright themes she created after viewing the photographs in the Warhol exhibit. For the rest of her life, Audrey credited Warhol with her success because had she not seen his gallery show, she might never have changed her style.

Andy Warhol first displayed his Campbell's soup cans and other commercialized paintings at the Ferus Gallery on July 9, 1962.

7. Touch a Star

Lina stood along Hollywood Boulevard, her eyes taking in all the noises and sights around her. She was on the corner of Gower, watching a group of workmen bent over a section of the sidewalk. She walked over to see what they were doing.

A bronze and gold star was placed in a square on the sidewalk, emblazoned with the name "Stanley Kramer." Lina's eyes grew large as she knew who that was. She remembered sitting in the movie theater watching his films *On the Beach* and *The Defiant Ones*. These films made her decide acting was her passion and led her to come to Los Angeles to fulfill that dream.

"What is this for?" she asked the workers.

"They are constructing a Hollywood Walk of Fame," one of the men said. "This guy gets the first permanent star. Next week, we will install them for Joanne Woodward, Burt Lancaster, and Edward Sedgwick. I think they are planning a ceremony to unveil Joanne Woodward's."

Lina was excited to hear that more stars would be installed. She asked the men what day the ceremony would be and was told February 9.

On the morning of February 9, Lina dressed in her most excellent outfit and returned to Hollywood Boulevard. She stood among the crowd to see Joanne Woodward get the first official star on the Walk of Fame. A tarp covered the star, although Lina knew what it would look like having seen the one for Stanley Kramer.

The crowd cheered as Joanne Woodward and her husband, Paul Newman, walked through the public to the star. The couple posed for photos before Joanne pulled the tarp from the star, revealing the gold and brass display with her name emblazoned across the top. She sat with her feet to the side, her striped dress spread around her as photographers snapped the photos.

Lina clapped along with the rest of the crowd as the couple was ushered away.

“Someday, my name will be on one of those stars,” Lina said.

Lina’s dream came true when she earned a star on the Hollywood Walk of Fame for directing almost 30 years later.

The Hollywood Walk of Fame held their official groundbreaking on February 8, 1960.

8. Time for Lunch

Elmer walked through the Woolworths store, picking up the few needed items. As he circled the store, he noticed the four young black men in jackets and ties also picking up random things in the store.

Elmer decided to take a break from running errands and enjoy a piece of pie before he headed home. He wandered into the lunch counter area and sat at the counter.

A few moments later, the four young black men walked into the lunch counter area, causing a few looks from other diners. In 1960, it was illegal for blacks to sit in the lunch counter area in North Carolina.

Elmer heard one of the men place an order, but he was refused. Elmer listened to the young man as he responded.

“But we are customers here,” the young man said, pulling a receipt out of his pocket to show he had just purchased items in the store.” We've already purchased items today, and we can prove it. We’ve got receipts. We bought all these things here, and we just want to be served.”

Elmer began to feel sympathy for the young men, realizing that the four men had done nothing wrong and had spent money in the store before coming to the counter.

Suddenly, a police officer entered the store and walked behind the young men. He said nothing but paced back and forth behind them, smacking his billy club in his hand. Elmer began to feel angry as he realized that the four young men were being threatened with physical harm simply because they were black and sitting in a “white’s only” area. He was impressed that the young men held their ground, not resorting to violence or cowering.

An older customer came over and sat beside the four young men, telling them she was disappointed in their actions. When asked why, she said she was disappointed they had not done it sooner.

The older woman’s comments resonated with Elmer; he knew it was time for whites to step up. A few days later, he joined students from several schools and colleges in the area. He was one of a few white people standing in with the blacks who were simply asking to eat lunch at Woolworths.

Several months later, Elmer stood proudly in the Woolworths restaurant and watched three black women removed their aprons and were the first served at the counter, effectively ending segregation in a small North Carolina department store.

On February 1, 1960, Joseph McNeil, Franklin McCain, David Richmond, and Jibreel Khazan sat at a Woolworth's lunch counter in Greensboro, North Carolina, effectively starting a movement that was the first step toward desegregation in the southern states.

9. The Mayor of Olympic Village

Joe looked around in awe at the sights of the Olympic Village in Rome. He was there as a photographer's assistant and had gotten a rare afternoon off to explore independently. As he turned a corner, Joe saw a young man walking toward him. Joe stopped as he watched the young man shake hands with everyone he met.

"Who is that guy?" Joe asked someone next to him.

"That is Cassius Clay," the man replied. "I read he is favored to win the gold in boxing, but I've never even heard of him."

Each day, as Joe and his boss wandered around Olympic Village taking photos, they saw the young man talking to everyone he met, shaking hands, and introducing himself. Joe was excited to watch the man box in his opening round.

In that round, Joe watched as the referee stopped the fight in the second round and, a few days later, watched as he beat a Russian boxer. Clay won his next contest sending him to the finals.

In the final round, Joe knew that Clay was up against a powerhouse from Russia and was not expected to win.

As soon as Clay stepped into the ring, though, Joe felt the shift in the crowd. The Mayor of the Olympic Village took control, and it seemed they were behind the young man. Initially, the fight looked very mismatched as Clay seemed to struggle with the southpaw style of the Russian. His fancy footwork, which had served him so well to this point, became a hindrance, so by the third round, he shifted his tactic. He stopped relying on his footwork and threw hard punches instead.

The fight continued, and by the final round, Clay had found his rhythm, striking harder and more precisely until the Russian was dazed. At the end of the match, the Russian was slumped against the ropes, and no question had won.

Joe's boss snapped photos of the medal round with Cassius Clay standing tall and strong with a gold medal around his neck. The silver medalist, the Russian he had just beaten, stood next to him, blood still on his shirt. Two men tied for the bronze medal, and stood on the other side of the 18-year-old Clay.

One thing Joe knew after watching the young man box was that a great athlete had just been introduced to the world.

Cassius Clay, who later became Muhammed Ali, won the gold medal at the 1960 Olympic Games in Rome.

10. The Debate That Changed Politics

Edward and Margaret sat down in their living room. Dinner was over, the kitchen cleaned up, and the children bathed and tucked into bed. Edward turned on the television before dropping into his recliner. Margaret picked up her knitting needles as the ABC News commentators began to speak.

“We are waiting for the two candidates to take the stage,” the announcer said. “This is a moment in history since it is the first time the American people will be able to watch a presidential debate from the comfort of their own homes.”

The camera switched to show Vice-President Richard M. Nixon walking onto the stage. He was limping slightly.

“I guess his knee is still giving him problems,” Edward said.

“Poor thing,” Margaret said, shaking her head. “He did just get out of the hospital. Goodness, he looks awfully pale, too. Maybe he should have rescheduled this.”

Just as she said that Margaret saw Senator John F. Kennedy take the stage.

“He is such a handsome man,” she said, laying her knitting in her lap. “I don’t understand why people think he will lose this election.”

Edward laughed.

“Margaret, you don’t vote for someone because they are handsome,” he said. “Did you hear about the speech Nixon made back in 1952, and how about that debate with Khrushchev?”

“I know, dear, but didn’t Kennedy win the debate against Humphrey recently?” she said, picking up her knitting again. “And, honestly, he looks so much healthier than Nixon.”

Edward and Margaret watched as Howard K. Smith moderated the debate between the two candidates.

“We can no longer afford to be second best. I want people all over the world to look to the United States again, to feel that we’re on the move, to feel that our high noon is in the future,” Kennedy said, causing Margaret to put down her knitting again.

The couple listened as the two men went back and forth, with many questions about Kennedy’s experience and what Nixon had done as vice president. When the debate ended, Edward looked over at Margaret.

“I really think Jack Kennedy answered the questions best,” Edward said. “He might be more than just a pretty face.”

Margaret smiled, knowing that the debate might have encouraged her husband to vote for the young, reasonably unknown senator over the polished vice-president in the election a few months later.

The first televised presidential debate was held on September 26, 1960, and many say that the debate changed the political landscape.

11. The Power of Women

Cheryl stomped upstairs to her room and slammed the door. Her father had just told her that she was a girl and should have no opinion on things of the world.

"If you go to college, you will become a nurse or a teacher," her father said one night over dinner. "I am not paying for you to get a degree you will never use. Once you meet a guy, you will just get married."

It was 1965, and Cheryl knew that the world was changing. She had checked out Betty Friedan's *The Feminine Mystique* from the local library, learning that women should have opportunities beyond traditional roles as mothers and housewives. The book opened Cheryl's eyes to the fact that there was a world out there that she wanted to explore. She tried expressing it to her mother.

One day, while wandering through the library, Cheryl found a book called *Sex and the Single Girl* by someone named Helen Gurley Brown. Cheryl recalled a movie that starred Natalie Wood the same name, but her parents refused to let her see it when it was in the theater. She checked out the book and took it home, hiding it among her schoolbooks and reading it at night under her covers.

The book opened Cheryl's eyes to a world she never knew existed. The book proved to her that she could be financially independent and that she did not need to rely on a husband to have money. Although there was a lot about sex before marriage in the book and tips on finding the right man, the chapters on climbing to the top of the business world, decorating an apartment, and living a life of independence resonated with Cheryl.

The day after finishing the book, Cheryl visited her high school guidance counselor and informed her that she wanted to attend college. She explained her dilemma: her father would not cover the cost unless she went into nursing or teaching.

Four years later, Cheryl graduated with a degree in English literature and obtained a job with a paper in New York. She spent the next 20 years traveling the world as a journalist and photographer with her husband. After retiring from the article, Cheryl took a position as a college professor, finally fulfilling her father's dream for her to become a teacher after pursuing her passion.

In 1962, Helen Gurley Brown published Sex and the Single Girl, while in 1963, Betty Friedan published The Feminine Mystique, igniting the women's movement.

12. Gateway to the West

John stood in the crowd, remembering when a time capsule, with signatures of hundreds of thousands of school children, was welded into the keystone as part of a project that had taken decades to complete. A native of St. Louis, John had been proud to be part of what had been dubbed the "topping out" ceremony of the Gateway Arch in 1965, a monument that would stand to welcome visitors into the great west and acknowledge the sacrifices of those who explored the land many years before.

He recalled a helicopter transporting Vice-President Hubert

Humphrey circled overhead as a priest and rabbi prayed over the keystone on that historic day. The final piece of the arch was about eight feet long and was installed at noon to complete the monument that John had watched develop over most of his life. John recalled how the final piece of the arch had been established.

Today, over three years later, on a rainy spring day, John stood in the crowd to see the dedication ceremony of the arch. He heard Vice-President Humphrey call the arch a "soaring curve in the sky that links the rich heritage of yesterday with the richer future of tomorrow," which John agreed was true.

One of the main reasons that John was so pleased to be part of this ceremony was that it had provided him with a new lease on life. Unemployed for several months after his company shut down, he would begin work at the nearby visitor center. John knew that the arch would revitalize the riverfront area, a place that had fallen into disrepair but now had a new lease on life, just as he did.

As Vice-President Humphrey concluded his speech, John felt a surge of pride as he looked at the big silver arch. He recalled his grandparents, who told stories of their travels into the western part of the United States, where they entered the fur trade. Seeing the turn welcoming everyone to this area of the country made John incredibly proud of his heritage.

The Gateway Arch in St. Louis had been planned since 1933. It was completed in 1965, with an opening ceremony in 1968.

13. Into the Deep

Standing on the ship's bow, Steven felt the ocean's wind in his face. Steven, a ship engineer, felt that he was about to be part of history as he watched the submersible ship pulled from the ocean with Don Walsh and Jacques Piccard inside.

The crew had been practicing for this day for months off the coast of Guam, taking the submersible craft deeper and deeper to test it. The *Trieste* had performed admirably, and decided to take it to the deepest part of the ocean, the Challenger Deep in the Mariana Trench. The submersible had travelled 24,000 feet below the sea surface just over a week earlier with no issues. It had been determined that January 23, 1960, would be the day to see if she could survive in the deepest part of the ocean. The mission had succeeded, and Steven could not wait to hear what Piccard and Walsh had seen.

The two men climbed out of the submersible onto the ship to applause from the crew. The excited crew and engineers surrounded them and questions flew at them. It had taken them over four hours to get to the bottom of the ocean and over three hours to return to the ship. They could communicate while down there, something that surprised both the men in the submersible and the engineers.

“We stirred the bottom sediment, which is very fine and granular,” Walsh said to the crew. “There was no way to photograph anything because it felt like we were sitting in a bowl of milk. The current didn’t move it away like normal, which was strange.”

“Just before we landed, we saw what looked like a halibut, sole or flounder, about a foot long," Piccard said. "We were shocked as we did not expect to see fish that deep in the ocean, but we could not be sure what type of fish it was."

Steven knew that he had just witnessed history in the making and that undersea exploration would never be the same. Over the next few years, he helped the crew with different modifications to the *Trieste,* exploring the Atlantic Ocean, off the coast of New England, and in many other areas of the world.

The Trieste made its maiden voyage to the deepest part of the ocean on January 23, 1960.

14. A Big Show

In 1964, Debbie's parents gave her tickets to the Ed Sullivan Show for her birthday. Living close to New York, she had always wanted to be in the studio audience for the show on which so many famous people appeared. Debbie and her parents traveled to the studio on February 9 for the show and were shocked to see all the security guards on site.

"I wonder who is on the show tonight?" said Debbie's mother.

"I heard it is some new band out of England," her father said. "Maybe they protect singers more over there than we do."

Debbie's eyes lit up as she knew the "new" band her father mentioned was The Beatles. She had been listening to their album for weeks but had no idea they would be appearing on Ed Sullivan the night she and her parents had tickets for the show.

The three of them progressed through the security, with Debbie's parents having to show their tickets along the way. Any young person was stopped and questioned unless they had an adult with them. They found their seats in the studio while Debbie tried to remain calm, but the girl behind her began to scream.

The entire audience erupted into screams as the band took the stage, opening with "All My Loving" before moving into "Till There Was You" and then "She Loves You." The audience screamed the entire time as the four men played their set. When they finished, the show went to a commercial break before Sullivan returned to the stage. He tried to quiet the crowd and introduced a magician. Charlie Brill and Mitzi McCall attempted to do a funny skit, but the crowd was so loud Debbie could hardly hear them talk.

Finally, Ed Sullivan brought the Beatles back on the stage, where they sang "I Want to Hold Your Hand" and "I Saw Her Standing There" as the crowd went wild. Debbie could not contain herself and began screaming along with everyone else, standing in front of her chair and dancing.

On the ride home, Debbie could not stop talking about the Beatles. She played their album repeatedly until her parents begged her to stop. Her mother even bought their newest album so that she could hear different songs. From that day forward, Debbie was a diehard Beatles fan who attended many concerts and even met some band members as an adult.

The Beatles made their television debut on The Ed Sullivan Show on February 9, 1964.

15. Equal Rights for All

Sherri was the first person in her family to attend college, so she was thrilled when she got into UC Berkeley. Her first year, 1963, had been eye-opening as she realized that things were much different at this unique higher learning institute than in her small town in rural Kentucky. This was Sherri's first exposure to varying opinions on race, gender, and the world itself.

In September of her sophomore year, Sherri joined several of her friends at what was supposed to be a rally for civil rights at a local Sheraton. When they arrived, they discovered that thousands were arguing that more black individuals should be in executive positions. Most of those present were students from Berkeley. She recognized many students from her classes.

Sherri was not pleased with the reaction from the Sheraton when the group pushed for equal rights. As a political science major, Sherri decided she wanted to be involved in the fight for equality. A few weeks later, all students received a letter stating that political gatherings were now prohibited on the corner of Bancroft and Telegraph, where Sherri had spent considerable time with others pushing political matters.

A few days later, Sherri and other members of the Congress of Racial Equality (CORE) set up a table in front of Sproul Hall, a popular gathering place for students. Sherri was supposed to be handling the table the afternoon of October 1, 1964. She was on her way to do so when she learned the president of CORE had been arrested for violating a policy against political activism. Sherri and her friends were enraged and headed to the hall quickly.

They arrived to find Jack in the back of a police car. Sherri and many other students sat down in the street, preventing the police car from leaving. Throughout the night, students gave speeches while standing on the vehicle as a crowd of thousands gathered to watch. The next day, an agreement was reached between the administration and students regarding political speech on campus.

The sit-in at Sproul Hall led Sherri to a lifetime of activism. She fought for the rights of people of color and women and was recognized for her activism throughout her life.

In the fall of 1964 and into 1965, students conducted several sit-ins in an effort to promote equal rights at UC Berkeley and to protest actions by the university to quell student activism.

16. A Clothing Rebellion

Jessica walked down the street in London, happy to have a day off from the office. As an American working in the city, she enjoyed learning more about British culture and was excited to have a free afternoon to explore.

She walked past a cute little boutique and stopped quickly. On the mannequin was the shortest skirt she had ever seen. She glanced at the sign on the boutique and raised her eyebrows.

“Bazaar,” she said to herself. “This is kind of bizarre, for sure.”

Jessica strolled into the small store and walked over to a rack of tiny skirts. She pulled one out and looked at it. The girl who had been behind the counter walked over to her.

"Isn't that just lovely?" she said, her accent thick. "We just got them in the store, and they seem to be so popular. Our owner calls them the "mini." Funny story, she named it after her favorite car!"

Jessica carried one of the skirts to the dressing room and tried it on. It hit her just a few inches below her bottom, revealing her leg well above her knee. It felt freeing as she turned to look at herself in the mirror. Impulsively, she purchased the skirt, carrying it to the counter.

"This is so exciting!" the girl said as she bagged the skirt. "I think you will just love it."

Jessica was meeting friends the next day for dinner, so she decided to wear the cute little skirt she just bought. She arrived at the restaurant to find her friends waiting outside.

"Jessica!" her friend, Louise, said. "That skirt!"

"Isn't it just perfect!" Jessica said, twirling around before Louise grabbed her arm.

"You better stop, or you are going to flash your knickers at everyone," Louise said, laughing. Jessica laughed as well as she, Louise, and Claudine walked into the restaurant.

Jessica returned to the little boutique and bought several more of the tiny skirts over the next few weeks, finding that she felt bold, feminine, and attractive in the tiny dresses that showed so much leg.

Louise and Claudine had also purchased a few of the little skirts within a few weeks. It made Jessica happy to have been ahead of the new trend when she bought the little dress from the boutique she just happened to wander by.

Mary Quant introduced her version of the miniskirt at her London boutique, Bazaar, in 1964, creating a fashion trend that would last for decades.

17. The Big Game

"Hurry up, Dad; the game is about to start!" Billy said, pulling on his father's hand as they climbed the stadium steps. Billy and his father had traveled to Los Angeles from their small town of Lisbon, Wisconsin, to watch their beloved Green Bay Packers play the Kansas City Chiefs in the first-ever NFL championship game.

"This is going to be the best game ever," Billy said as they returned to their seats. Billy could see everything, even though they were high up in the stands. The Packers had only lost two games all year, but the Chiefs had only lost two, with one game ending in a tie.

Billy could see Vince Lombardi standing on the sidelines and clapping as Bart Starr walked out on the field. The game was exciting, even though the Chiefs seemed to rule the first half, despite the Packers scoring the first touchdown. At halftime, the score was so close Billy was worried his Packers would lose.

In the third quarter, however, Willie Wood intercepted a pass and ran to the five-yard line, where Mike Garrett tackled him. On the very next play, Elijah Pitts scored, causing Billy and his father to yell and clap as the score put the Packers solidly in the lead. Pitts scored again in the fourth quarter, and the Packers won 35 to 10.

“I can’t believe I saw Fred Williamson get knocked out in that game,” Billy gushed as he and his father exited the stadium. “And then he broke his arm! This was the best day ever!”

Billy remained a lifelong Packers fan, never forgetting when his father took him to the first Superbowl in 1967.

The first Superbowl was played January 15, 1967.

18. Yale’s Superwomen

The *New York Times* labeled her a “superwoman,” a title that Becky did not think applied. She was sitting at home in Chicago, waiting to learn if she would be accepted to Yale, where she would be among the first women ever to attend the all-male Ivy League college. If she did not get into Yale, she would be satisfied with attending the University of Chicago that fall, something she was mentally prepared to do. A few days after the article in *The Times*, Becky learned she would be one of four women attending Yale in the fall.

“I don’t feel like a superwoman,” Becky thought to herself, a sentiment the other three women also felt.

On the bus from the airport, Becky met two young men wearing Yale jackets who offered to help her carry her bags to the dorm on the top floor of Vanderbilt Hall. She overheard one of the male students comment that Yale would never be the same. When she glanced at him, she realized he was smiling, and knew he felt that this change was good.

Challenges appeared immediately, but some were amusing. The bathrooms at Vanderbilt Hall had been retrofitted for women, but the mirrors were placed too high on the wall for most women to use them. The administration was also very apologetic about the lack of bathtubs, and the four women joked that maybe administrators were unaware that women could shower. Becky got another surprise when she appeared at the swimming pool for a required swimming test to see a sign that said, "Clothing must now be worn in public places." She asked about the character and was told that men used to perform the test naked. Doors were so heavy the women sometimes needed both arms to open them.

Becky felt the need to prove herself as men significantly outnumbered women at the university. She and the women she roomed with worked hard to clarify that they were there as students, not potential wives.

Becky's four years at Yale were fruitful; she graduated with a degree in fine arts. She eventually married and earned an MBA.

Yale began admitting women in 1968, later than many of the Ivy League universities.

19. Turn On, Tune In or Drop Out

Standing in Golden Gate Park, Valerie was embracing her new freedom. Deciding that college was not for her, she had left her small town in rural Pennsylvania and hitchhiked her way to the San Francisco area, much to the dismay of her parents. For the past few months, she had worked in a small coffee shop, living in a home with six other people to save on living expenses.

One of her roommates had told her about the "Human Be-In" at the park. Since arriving in the Bay Area, Valerie had learned a lot about the free spirit life. For the first time, she had experimented with psychedelics and was enjoying the communal lifestyle with friends who didn't live the staid, quiet life she was used to back East.

Valerie listened as Timothy Leary spoke to the crowd, telling them to "turn on, tune in, drop out," and the comment resonated with her. She was surrounded by people in bright colors and women wearing flowing dresses with flowers in their hair. The atmosphere was charged with a feeling of freedom and relaxation.

Over the next few months, Valerie immersed herself in the hippie culture, especially as the coffee shop in Haight-Asbury began to cater to the underground crowd. Poets and musicians began to perform there, leading her to develop a keen appreciation for their talents.

Throughout that summer, Valerie embraced the free-spirit lifestyle. Many of those who joined her in the San Francisco area left at the end of the summer, returning to school or getting full-time jobs. Valerie remained, eventually purchasing the coffee shop and turning it into a location where young musicians started, building a lucrative career based on the Summer of Love.

The Summer of Love was a social phenomenon in the Haight-Asbury neighborhood near San Francisco and is credited with creating the hippie counterculture of the 1960s.

20. The First Pony Car

Ralph stopped short as he passed the dealership, noticing the car in the window. He had never seen a car that was so unique. He wandered into the showroom, walked over to the car, and was surprised to see the price tag was less than $3,000.

“That is our new Ford Mustang,” a salesman said as he walked over. “She’s a beauty, isn’t she?”

Ralph grinned and nodded. He asked why the car was so reasonably priced, and the salesman explained that it was designed using parts found in other Ford models. He told Ralph they had one outside if he wanted to take a test drive.

Ralph and the salesman hopped into the car and took off from the dealership. The car ran smoothly but had a sporty feel that Ralph liked. He especially liked the downward-sloping section from the roof to the trunk, something the salesman called a fastback. He loved the clean lines and their ease of handling.

They returned to the lot, and Ralph sat down to talk to the salesman. They negotiated a price for a stunning Arcadian Blue model on the showroom floor. Once all the documents were signed, Ralph headed home in his new car.

He pulled into the driveway, and his mother came out, wiping her hands on her apron.

“What is that?” she asked. “I didn’t know you were planning to buy a car.”

Ralph explained that he happened to be walking by the showroom, and this car caught his eye. He told her what he paid, and her eyes grew big. She told him he was crazy for buying such a fancy car and headed into the house even at that price.

Later that evening, Ralph headed for a drive, pulling into his favorite hangout. His friends were in awe of his new Arcadian Blue Mustang, all asking for rides in the fun car.

Several years later, Ralph married, and his wife begged him to sell the car when they had children, but he refused. He knew that the 1965 Mustang he bought on a whim was a classic, and he was correct. More than 20 years later, Ralph handed the keys to his son, who still drives it today.

The Ford Mustang was introduced at the 1964 World’s Fair, becoming an iconic automobile almost immediately.

Welcome to the 70s

1. Video Game Savior

Jason sat in his doctor's office. The cast on his arm was heavy. He had fallen again, and his mother was becoming worried. This was his third broken bone in five years, and at 17, he was tired of constantly finding out he had suffered another injury.

Dr King sat down on the little stool in the exam room and slid over in front of Jason. He looked over the cast, asked Jason to wiggle his fingers, and then sat back. He opened the file and read something before closing it and placing it on the exam table.

"Jason, I think there is more to this than clumsiness," Dr. King said. "I actually think you have something called spatial awareness disorder. I just want to ask you a few questions to confirm the diagnosis."

The doctor asked questions and then looked at Jason's mother.

"This is going to sound crazy, but there is something I think you need to do," Dr. King said. "There is a company that just released a game console. It is for playing video games on your TV at home. It is called Atari, and I think you need to invest in one."

Jason's eyes lit up. He had been begging his mother to get him an Atari console since they were released the year before. He laughed at the expression on his mother's face as she questioned the doctor. Dr King continued, saying that the games had shown promise in helping kids with spatial awareness disorder. On the way home that afternoon, Jason and his mother purchased the console at the store. His mother was not pleased with the cost but felt she was willing to try if it would help Jason with his clumsiness.

For the next few months, Jason played the Atari almost every day. Eventually, he felt like he was more coordinated, and his falls seemed to stop. Finally, Jason upgraded his consoles, expanding his gaming systems significantly. At college, he developed an interest in creating games himself and earned his degree in the computer engineering department. After graduation, he landed a job with an up-and-coming video game company, eventually rising to upper management and leaving his spatial disorder issues behind.

The Atari 2600 game console was released in 1977, marking the beginning of the at-home video game phenomenon.

2. May the Force Be with You

Judy and Claire paid their admission to the movie theater, heading in to watch the new movie that had just come to their small town. It was 1978, and everyone was talking about the movie *Star Wars*. Living in a small town, they often had to wait several months before new movies arrived, and this was the feature for the week at their small movie theater. The two women worked together in a local doctor's office and often hung out on weekends. They were both skeptical of this movie but figured there was so much of a buzz about it. They just had to see what everyone was talking about.

"I thought this was about the future," Judy whispered as the movie began with a rolling text about the past. "This sounds like it happened a long time ago." Claire nodded, her eyes glued to the screen. Suddenly, a space battle begins, and the two women jump.

They watched as the giant spaceship dwarfed the smaller spacecraft that must carry the princess.

Both Judy and Claire were hooked from that moment. It took quite some time for the hero, Luke Skywalker, to appear, but they knew as soon as they saw him that he was someone to watch. They laughed at the antics of Han Solo and his sidekick, Chewy, and C3PO and R2D2. Judy and Claire could not wait to tell their friends when the movie ended.

A few weeks later, Judy was having lunch with her mother when the subject of *Star Wars* came up. Judy was shocked to learn that her mother loved the film as well. The two of them began conversing about what the movie meant to them. Judy also found that her younger brother was a fan, and she marveled at how one film had appealed to multiple generations in such a way.

Over the years, Judy, her mother, and her brother bonded over their love for a little film with a powerful message. Little did Judy know that when she went to the movies that Saturday night with her friend, Claire, what she saw would change her life and bring her closer to her family.

The first movie, Star Wars: A New Hope, was released in 1977 and became a box office sensation as well as a cult classic.

3. What to Wear

Lydia had never been to a disco, but a group from her office had decided to visit one on a Saturday night. She was digging through her closet, finding nothing that would work. Most of her clothes were for work, blazers, fitted blouses, and skirts she wore with high heels. She knew they would not work on her night out. She grabbed her purse and headed to the mall.

"I have the perfect thing for you," one salesgirl said when Judy wandered in and told her what she needed. "These just came in this week, so few people have seen them yet." The girl went in the back and came out with a dress different from anything Lydia had ever seen. It was made of a soft jersey material, and instead of a typical dress that was pulled over the head, this one slid on like a jacket with a belt that held it closed. The neckline was lower than anything Lydia had worn before.

She took it into the dressing room to try it on and was shocked to see that it fit her like a glove. She loved the way the dress hugged her curves, the dress accentuated the curve of her hips, and the material was very comfortable. She exited the dressing room and told the girl she would take it. She headed back into the mall, where she saw a pair of shoes in a perfect window. She purchased them and headed home.

On Saturday, she wore her new dress and shoes, and then called a cab to take her to the club. She arrived just as a few of her friends did and was pleased with the compliments she got on her outfit. Inside the club, they found a table and ordered drinks. The music was loud, and it did not take long for them to hit the dance floor. Lydia received lots of attention in her new dress and immediately knew she needed to upgrade her style.

The next day, she revisited the mall, purchasing a tube top, spandex shorts, some wide-legged pants, and a few tops with glitter. She began to be a regular at the club, dancing the night away. It was at the club where she met Bill, and the two began meeting there regularly. Bill recalled her first night at the club wearing the wrap dress. Lydia was surprised he would remember, but he told her she was stunningly beautiful in the dress.

One year later, Bill and Lydia were married. Lydia was sure to pack the wrap dress in her suitcase for the honeymoon.

The 1970s ushered in a new era in clothing, including bell-bottom jeans, midi skirts, tube tops, and jersey wrap dresses.

4. Immaculate Reception

Carl was excited to have tickets to the playoff game between his beloved Pittsburgh Steelers and the Oakland Raiders. It had been difficult in his hometown of Pittsburgh, as the steel industry seemed to be declining. The only exciting thing was that the city's adored NFL team was in the playoffs and the game promised to be good.

Carl took his seat, happy he was not far from the 50-yard line even though he was high up in the stands. His brother, Calvin, sat next to him, and they both talked about how they felt this team could go to the big game.

The game proved to be a nail-biter in the first half. Carl and Calvin screamed when John Fuqua came close to scoring, only to be stopped when Jack Tatum tackled him.

"Why didn't they take the field goal?" Carl cried, plopping down in his seat after the fourth and two runs.

The half ended with no score, and the brothers wandered to a concession stand for food. They returned to their seats, eagerly awaiting the rest of the game. Pittsburgh scored a field goal in the first possession, drawing first blood. Carl and Calvin screamed again when the Oakland quarterback was intercepted by Jack Ham, leading the coach to put in a new quarterback.

The following Oakland possession was not a happy moment for Carl and Calvin when Oakland scored a touchdown and extra point, giving them a seven-to-six lead.

“There is only about a minute left,” Calvin said, disgustedly tossing his hat in his lap. Carl told him to have faith as the next play began.

Carl’s hopes faded as the Steelers got nowhere on the field. With 22 seconds left at their 40-yard line, the brothers felt like they were about to watch their beloved team get knocked out of the playoffs.

Suddenly, Bradshaw dropped back and, under pressure, threw the ball toward Fuqua. Just as the ball reached him, Fuqua collided with Jack Tatum, sending the ball backwards several yards. Carl and Calvin began screaming as Franco Harris picked up the ball and ran down the field, getting blocks and stiff-arming opponents into the end zone. The ensuing extra point gave the Steelers their first playoff win, thanks to Harris’ fantastic catch.

The Immaculate Reception is the name given to one of the most famous plays in NFL history that took place on December 23, 1972.

5. Celebrating Earth

Kimberly called out to get her students' attention as they sat at their desks. Over the past few weeks, the class has been learning about the environment and how they could protect the Earth. A few months earlier, Kimberly listened to a speech by Senator Gaylord Nelson, who had put together an environmental initiative. She felt that the ecological "teach-ins" he was planning would be a great way to help her young students learn about protecting the environment.

To see how she could use the senator's ideas in her classroom, Kimberly had written to the senator, explaining that she taught fourth grade and felt it was the perfect age to begin instilling a love of the Earth into her students. She had received a response from his office telling her that national activities were planned on April 22, 1970, and providing her with a list of ideas for her classroom. One suggestion was to plant trees and perform cleanups in the community.

After discussing with her principal, Kimberly decided to buy ten saplings for the day. The principal permitted for her to plant the trees on a small patch of ground on the other side of the playground. Kimberly was excited to tell her students what they would be doing.

"Today, we are going to put our ideas about how to help the Earth into action," Kimberly told them. "We have ten trees, and I have collected some shovels that we are going to use to dig holes and plant them by the playground. Since there are 30 of you and ten trees, you will work in groups of three, so let's count off by three."

To the students, Kimberly knew this was a fun day out of the classroom, but her goal was that each of them would understand the importance of trees in the environment. While outside, she walked around to each group, lending a hand when they needed it and asking them what they were learning. They all mentioned different things, from the worms and bugs they found as they dug to the size of the saplings that would eventually grow to be large trees.

Years later, when Kimberly would go outside the school or even just drive by, those ten trees symbolised what she had done on the first Earth Day.

The first Earth Day was held April 22, 1970, just eight months before the establishment of the Environmental Protection Agency (EPA).

6. The King Says Aloha

Michael and Lisa could hardly contain their excitement. Elvis fans since they were both young, especially since Lisa's full name was Lisa Marie. After the singer's daughter, the couple was at home with their children, preparing them for bed. Lisa was finishing their baths while Michael opened a bottle of wine, preparing to settle in and watch the King perform live from Hawaii.

Since Colonel Tom Parker announced that Elvis would perform in Hawaii, Michael and Lisa followed the story closely. They were disappointed when it was decided not to air the concert live because it would compete with the Super Bowl when it was aired in other countries. When it was announced it would air in April instead, the couple decided to make it a "date night" at home in front of the television set.

"Both our little darlings are in bed," Lisa said, walking down the stairs. She smiled when she saw the wine glasses and bottle on the table. "Well, this looks like a promising evening."

Michael laughed and hugged his wife, kissing her on the forehead.

"It is not often I get a date night with you, even if it is at home watching Elvis," he laughed. The two settled on the sofa, and Michael poured each a glass of wine just as the concert began.

Elvis looked handsome in his white suit with a bald eagle emblazoned. Lisa commented that he looked as if he was slimmer than he had been the last time they had seen him on television. The performance was electrifying, and the couple danced around the living room to some of their favorites, including "Blue Suede Shoes" and "Hound Dog." They slowly danced to "Can't Help Falling in Love," a song played at their wedding.

As the show ended, Lisa clapped as Elvis threw his belt into the crowd and again after he threw a cape he was wearing into the audience. Soon after, the concert ended.

"I think that was well worth waiting for," Michael said, gathering the wine glasses and empty bottle. He carried them to the kitchen as Lisa turned off the lights. They headed to bed, knowing they had just watched a legend perform.

Elvis Presley performed his show "Aloha from Hawaii," which was broadcast live in Asia and Oceania on January 14, 1973, but in the United States on April 4 of that year.

7. Don't Call Me Mrs.

The airport was crowded, and Diane rushed to the gate to check in for her flight. She could relax once she had provided the gate agent with her information. She still had about two hours before they would start boarding, so she decided to grab something to eat and pick up reading material for the plane. She stopped first at a small newsstand by her gate and headed to the magazine rack.

There, sitting mixed in with well-known publications like *Ladies Home Journal* and *Family Circle,* was one that had just one word as the title — *Ms.* Diane had heard the term before from women who were tired of being called Miss or Mrs.. At the same time, men were always known as Mr. She understood the frustration as it appeared women had to announce their marital status while men did not. She picked up a copy of the magazine and thumbed through it.

What she saw was surprising. The magazine's inside was filled with articles geared toward women's rights and minimal emphasis on men. She immediately headed to the counter to purchase a copy. While sitting in the airport bar with a martini and a sandwich, Diane began reading. The magazine spoke to her, especially since she was a woman trying to make it in a career that was male-dominated.

Diane immediately filled out the card to purchase a subscription and dropped it in a mailbox she saw outside the bar. On the plane, she continued to read, realizing that this magazine spoke to her as a female and heightened her desire to fight for women's rights.

After her business trip, Diane reached out to a local feminist group. She was very thankful that she had married a man with the same viewpoints as her, and Eric was very supportive. Over the years, Diane became heavily involved in women's rights, raising her sons to be feminists. Many years later, her daughters-in-law thanked her for raising young men who understood women's plight and worked hard to make sure their wives and daughters were heard.

For the rest of her life, Diane was grateful that she stopped at that airport newsstand and picked up a copy of a magazine that changed the lives of many women.

The first issue of Ms Magazine was published July 1, 1972, and was the first periodical to focus on feminist news and information.

8. Walt's World

Sharon stood outside the gates of the new amusement park, her excitement evident. An avid Disney fan, she knew that she was about to witness history in the making. Sharon had visited Disneyland multiple times and loved the rides, the shows, and especially Sleeping Beauty's castle. Her mother joked when she was younger that Sharon thought the court was hers, while Sharon often told her mother she should be able to change her name to Aurora, Sleeping Beauty's real name.

Living in Florida and working at a local real estate office, Sharon could not get to Disneyland as often as she wanted. Over the past ten years, she has followed the story of the land purchases in the central Florida area. She was thrilled when an article was published in The Sentinel reporting that the land purchases were the first step in a new Disney Park. After Walt Disney passed away, Sharon was worried the park would never happen, but her hero's brother, Roy, carried on the legacy.

Today, that dream was becoming a reality. Sharon was among the first guests who would be entering the new park. When she entered the gates, she was instantly enamored of the attractions, realizing that this park would be far and away better than Disneyland. A few weeks later, she read that Roy Disney had named the park "Walt Disney World" in his brother's honor.

"Everyone has heard of Ford cars, but have they all heard of Henry Ford, who started it all," Roy had said. "Walt Disney World is named in memory of the man who started it all, so people will know his name as long as Walt Disney World is here." Sharon cried when Walt's widow, Lillian, said her husband would have been proud of the new park and cried again when Roy died less than three months after the park opened.

After the park opened, Sharon visited during a real estate convention. While there, she met an executive at the park who offered her a job in their real estate division. Sharon jumped at the chance to work for her favorite company and spent the next 20 years helping grow Walt Disney World into the attraction it is today.

Walt Disney World opened on October 1, 1971, the dream of Walt Disney, who passed away in 1966.

9. Golden Tickets

Dennis was bored as he strolled down the street. He had a rare weekend off from his restaurant job, but all his friends were working. Since they were all young, single, and living in a big city, this was not unusual, but Dennis simply did not want to sit at home on a Saturday afternoon.

He glanced up as he walked toward a theater and saw that there was a matinee of a new movie, *Willie Wonka and the Chocolate Factory*. He remembered a book he read as a boy about a young man and a chocolate factory and wondered if it was the same story. He saw the movie starred Gene Wilder, one of his favorite actors, so he decided to kill time and buy a ticket.

The movie begins with Charlie Bucket, the same child from the book he remembered reading when he was younger, who discovers a golden ticket to get into Willy Wonka's Chocolate Factory. He remembered characters from the book, including Augustus Gloop, Veruca Salt, Violet Beauregarde, and Mike Teevee.

The movie continues, and Dennis realizes it tells how character flaws can derail plans. When Charlie is thriving at the movie's end, Dennis realizes that it might be time for him to make some changes in his life.

Dennis leaves the movie theater and walks down the street to a small community college. The movie made him realise that he is wasting his life serving diners in a restaurant. Surprised that the admissions office was open on a Saturday, Dennis sat down with a counselor and discussed what he wanted out of life.

A month later, Dennis was sitting in his first college class, beginning a college career that would eventually earn him a doctorate in communication technology. After he married and had children, he had them watch the movie, explaining that their character says a lot about them and encouraging them always to do the right thing.

From the day he walked into that theater, Dennis credited Willy Wonka and the Chocolate Factory with changing his life.

10. Casting a Vote

Nancy sat in her car, unsure of what she needed to do. Just a few years before, President Richard M. Nixon had signed the 26th Amendment into law, allowing her to vote for the first time at 18. She recalled the fight to pass this, which was pushed through due to the war in Vietnam. Some of her high school classmates were over fighting the war, and since they were her age, she firmly agreed that they should have the right to vote. She also knew she had a responsibility to them to exercise that right.

Today, for the first time, Nancy would be voting for the president of the United States. Having turned 18 just a few months before, she had immediately registered to vote to have her voice heard. She had not discussed her presidential choice with her parents, although she had many discussions with her friends.

Gathering her nerve, Nancy climbed out of the car and walked inside the polling place. There was a short line, and she eventually made it to the table where they checked off her name and handed her a ballot to fill out in the voting booth. She walked inside and cast her vote, savoring the moment as a young teen who knew she was making history.

That night, Nancy sat on her parents' sofa and watched as Richard M. Nixon was elected for the second time. She hoped her vote made a difference as she did not feel his opponent was the right person for the job. From that day on, Nancy knew that she would always exercise her right to vote, realizing that men and women had died to give her that right. For the rest of her life, Nancy went to polling places every two years to vote, a habit she began soon after her 18th birthday.

On July 1, 1971, the 26th Amendment was ratified, lowering the voting age to 18.

11. Television and the Medic

It was quiet in the camp just before midnight as Gerald leaned back in the camp chair. The hospital tent was also quiet despite being full. Luckily, instead of those wounded in combat, the tent was full of soldiers with minor illnesses common during the adjustment to the different climates, creatures, and sicknesses in a foreign country.

Gerald looked up at the stars, still surprised at how vibrant they were in this foreign land. His career had taken him to many faraway places, and he had dealt with losses that he preferred not to consider. As a medic in the U.S. Army, Gerald treated soldiers with any number of illnesses and injuries, even though he served during a time of peace.

As he sat looking at the stars, Gerald remembered what led him to this career. As a child, he knew he wanted to enter the medical field after a cousin spent months in the hospital with an illness. He remembered his parents discussing how the doctors had "saved" his cousin. Since he had just realized he could not be an actual superhero like Spiderman, he decided that saving a life in a hospital was pretty close.

One night, he and his family sat down to watch television, and a new show came on called M*A*S*H. Gerald sat up as Hawkeye Pierce returned to his tent after time at the hospital tent operating on soldiers. Gerald and his family laughed while watching the antics of Hawkeye and his friend, Trapper John, and Margaret "Hot Lips" Houlihan, Frank Burns, and Colonel Henry Blake.

From that night on, Gerald was hooked on the television show that was part comedy, part drama. He felt sadness when Hawkeye or Trapper lost a patient. He laughed at the various problems they got themselves into and marveled at how they could skirt authority. Each season, Gerald's love of M*A*S*H grew, and he began to think about life as a military medic.

Gerald attended college and medical school, joining the U.S. Army immediately after. He had already spent a decade as a medic and knew this was his calling. He did learn quickly that the antics of Hawkeye and Trapper were fiction, but he still found that the medical professionals he worked with at the bases had their humorous way of dealing with the stressful job at hand. Sitting outside now, looking up, he thanked the stars that aligned, allowing him to live out the life he first saw on a unique television show when he was a child.

*The first episode of M*A*S*H was broadcast on September 17, 1972.*

12. The Great White

The weather in Martha's Vineyard was remarkable for a July day as Brian pulled into the parking lot of his hotel. This was a trip he had envisioned when he was a young boy, but not for the reasons most people believe. His career and this vacation were related to an event that happened when he was around 15 years old.

It was the summer of 1975, and Brian decided, along with a few friends, to go to the movies. *Jaws* was playing at the local theater, and they decided to see what all the hype was about. All of them were scary movie lovers, so this promised to be just another one that would scare them for a few hours, and they would move on.

Brian was hooked from the moment the movie began with its now iconic two-note opening theme. He was mesmerized as the shark attacked its victims and the ensuing drama that unfolded as the police chief and mayor fought to protect beachgoers. Brian was always interested in marine life and wondered if this was actually how a great white shark would act. He also wanted to know all he could about the filming of this outstanding movie.

Over the next few months, Brian devoured all the information he could about the movie *Jaws*. He learned that the town of Amity Island was Martha's Vineyard, and he vowed to go there one day. He also knew that the shark in the movie was mechanical and named "Bruce." He also learned that the story was loosely based on the true story of shark attacks 1916. Probably the most important thing he knew was that the film's portrayal of sharks as vengeful, spiteful murderers was false.

Soon after watching the movie, Brian announced to his family that he intended to become a marine biologist and hoped to focus his attention on sharks. He attended college and took a position on the East Coast, where he spent his days tracking sharks, using his knowledge to educate people on their mannerisms and movements.

Today, he was fulfilling his dream of walking on the beaches of “Amity Island,” the same beaches where many of the scenes were filmed. His only regret was that he would not be able to see “Bruce” swimming out among the breakers.

Jaws, based on a novel by Peter Benchley, was released in June 1975 and has become one of the most iconic movies of all time.

13. The Record Is Broken

The stadium was full as Jamar, and his father took their seats at the very top of the bleachers. They were in Atlanta and here to see their home team take on the Dodgers. Jamar knew he could see history made that day as his hero, Hank Aaron, had tied Babe Ruth’s record against the Cincinnati Reds earlier that week.

As a young black man, Jamar idolized how far Hank Aaron had come, along with Wily Mays and other players of color making strides in baseball. He felt that Hank was one of the best players on the Braves and prayed that he would see history be made that day.

The game reached the fourth inning without Hank sending one over the fence. Darrel Evans made it to first when Bill Russell committed an error. And then Hank stepped up to the plate.

"I have a good feeling about this," Jamar told his father, leaning forward in his seat.

The Dodgers' pitcher, Al Downing, who had walked Hank in the first inning, threw the first pitch, a ball. The stadium held its breath as the second pitch was thrown, a fastball up and over the plate. Jamar was out of his seat screaming before the ball even reached Hank, and the rest of the stadium erupted into screams as Hank swung, the ball sailing over the left field wall and into the Braves' bullpen.

Jamar and his father were jumping up and down, the entire stadium in an uproar. One of the Braves' pitchers appeared to catch the ball, but Jamar could not see past the jumping fans. He saw two young men run onto the field as Hank circled the bases, and the entire team surrounded him at home plate.

For more than 10 minutes, the crowd was out of control, screaming, jumping, and patting each other on the back. When everything died down and the game resumed, Jamar realized what he had just witnessed, someone who looked like him and had just broken the homerun record of a legend.

Henry "Hank" Aaron passed Babe Ruth's homerun record on April 8, 1974, when he hit his 715th homerun at his home stadium in Atlanta.

14. Where It Began

The room was finally clean, and Athena made her way back into the hotel hallway. She was exhausted as this was the tenth room she had cleaned in the past few hours, the 20th of the day. She always dreaded conventions at the hotel because most people who attended them made a mess of their rooms.

Despite only being 25, Athena felt like an older woman. She knew she was in a dead-end job and had no idea how to fix the problem as a black woman living in a big city. Her parents could not afford college, so she went to work immediately.

She arrived home to her tiny studio apartment and fixed her dinner. She carried the plate to the sofa and sat it on the small TV tray before walking over and turning on the black and white television on a little table across the room. Athena picked up her fork and sat down, waiting for the show she had anticipated.

The screen fills with a young black man running through a jungle. He is eventually caught and loaded on a ship bound for Maryland. Athena was hooked from the minute the series began. Every eight nights, Athena rushed home to watch the story of Kunta Kinte, Toby, and their families.

When the series ended, Athena knew she owed her ancestors something. She decided to begin researching her lineage to see if she could discover anything interesting. She became obsessed with genealogy and started saving her money to travel to exotic areas where she found connections.

One day, while on a break at work, she sat in the restaurant lobby, her books and papers spread out. An older gentleman walked over and asked her what she was doing. She explained she was researching her family history and trying to write short stories about her family. The man handed her a business card. He was an editor for a local paper.

"With the popularity of *Roots*, we are taking an interest in other African American stories," he told her. "Would you be interested in writing a column about your family and your discoveries?"

Athena jumped at the chance, and within a week, she had quit her job at the hotel to begin working on the paper. Eventually, Athena became one of the journalists at the paper, traveling around the world for stories and finally filling in the gaps in her lineage, thanks to the *Roots* documentary.

The Roots miniseries, based on a novel by Alex Haley, began airing on May 30, 2016, to almost instant critical acclaim.

15. Disco Life

Tina, Kelly, and Julie stood between the ropes outside the hottest club in town. The three women were dressed in the most stylish clothes of the day. Tina wore a skintight miniskirt with a glittery tube top. Kelly wore a striped jersey wrap dress, while Julie's minidress stopped just below her bottom and was adorned with glitter. All three had on high platform shoes, their hair curled, feathered away from their faces, and sprayed to keep it in place.

“I cannot believe we are about to get into this club!” Julie said as they moved forward in the line. Just two groups were ahead of them.

Within five minutes, they were inside and looking around in awe at the flashing lights, the glittering ball turning over their heads, and the dance floor that was pulsing and glowing. The DJ had not started yet, so the girls headed to the bar to get drinks and found a table.

Once they were seated, the music began. It was a thumping, base-laden song they all loved, so they made their way to the dance floor. The three women spent the following three pieces gyrating to the music and laughing with each other. Suddenly, a man with a name tag walked over to Kelly.

“I have been watching you dance,” he said. “We have a dance contest coming up in about 10 minutes. Would you like to be a contestant?”

Kelly was thrilled as she had spent her youth in dance classes. She agreed and moved to the bar to give the employee her information. Tina and Julie returned to their table where they could watch the contest.

The DJ announced the contest, and the competition began. Tina and Julie realized that Kelly had no match and were right. The judges chose her as the winner, telling her that no one else was anywhere near as good. Kelly returned to the table with a round of drinks, paying for them out of the $100 she had just won. The three women giggled and laughed, the two spectators congratulating Kelly on her win. Just then, another man walked up to the table. He handed Kelly his business card and introduced him as a talent agent. He asked her to give him a call the next day.

That night started a new career as a dancer for Kelly. She spent the next ten years as a backup dancer and then another 20 years as a choreographer, all because she decided to visit a disco.

Disco was both an extremely popular music genre and type of club and entertainment venue popular during the 1970s.

16. The Pope Has Been Chosen

Still mourning the loss of the leader of her church, Catherine was among the millions who awaited the plume of white smoke to indicate a successor had been chosen for Pope John Paul I, who had passed away just a month after being selected to lead the church. Sitting in her living room, folding laundry after her children had gone to bed, Catherine kept the television on to monitor the papal conclave constantly. Her husband was out in the garage, tinkering with an old car.

It had been three days, and Catherine, like Catholics around the world, was growing impatient to learn who would be chosen as the new leader. Born of Polish descent, she fully expected the new Pope to be Italian. She had heard that Cardinal Giuseppe Siri, the Archbishop of Genoa, and Cardinal Giovanni Benelli, Archbishop of Florence and a close friend of Pope John Paul I, were the frontrunners.

Suddenly, she heard an uproar from the crowd on television. She dropped the small shirt that she was folding in her lap and looked at the screen, which showed a white plume of smoke coming from the chimney of the Sistine Chapel, a clear indication there was now a new pope. Catherine was pleased she remembered the Latin she learned while attending Catholic schools when the announcement came across, even though there were subtitles.

"I announce to you a great joy. We have a Pope!" Catherine heard Cardinal Felici say. "The Most Eminent and Most Reverend Lord, Lord Karol Cardinal of the Holy Roman Church Wojtyla, who took himself the name John Paul."

Catherine's eyes welled with tears as she watched. Although it was clear that the news announcers had no idea who the new pope was, she was well aware. First, she knew he was not Italian but Polish, serving as the Archbishop of Krakow, a position he had held since 1967. She was thrilled he chose the name to honor his predecessor. John Paul I adopted the pontifical name of his two predecessors, Pope John XXIII and Pope Paul VI.

A few minutes later, the new pope appeared on the balcony and bestowed a blessing in Italian, not Latin, as was the custom.

"I have been called from a faraway land. If I make a mistake, please correct me," he said. "Praised by Jesus Christ! Dear brothers and sisters, we are still very saddened by the death of the very dear Pope John Paul I. And now, the most eminent cardinals have called a new bishop of Rome. They called from a far-away country, far, but always near in the communion of faith and the Christian tradition."

Catherine knew that the world would not be the same now that someone from the country where her ancestors originated was leading her church.

Pope John Paul II was chosen to lead the Catholic Church on October 16, 1978.

17. The Race That Changed a Sport

The snow had fallen overnight, and the world outside was buried in a blanket of white. Tim and his neighbor, Jeff, had spent the morning digging out sidewalks and driveways, trying to at least make a path to the road through the feet of snow that had fallen. Standing at the end of Tim's driveway, Jeff suggested they stop for the day as more snow was expected that evening, and he just remembered that the Daytona 500 would be aired on television that afternoon. Tim suggested Jeff and his wife come next door to watch the race as Tim's wife, Ellen, had a pot of chilli on the stove.

About an hour later, Jeff and his wife, Katie, arrived next door, with Katie carrying a basket of muffins she had baked earlier. The women headed to the kitchen while the men plopped in front of the television in the living room, sipping two beers. They groaned when they saw it had been raining and the track was wet.

"I sure hope they don't cancel this race," Jeff said. "I need a distraction from all that snow." A few minutes later, his wishes were granted, and the race began under caution. After 15 laps, the green flag was flashed, and the race started. Jeff and Tim were avid race fans and car junkies. They both attended stock car races up and down the East Coast, so watching a race on television was a thrill.

The race was exciting, with Buddy Baker pushed out early with engine trouble. Then, on lap 31, a tangle-up between Donnie Allison and Cale Yarborough added to the excitement. Although they all fell behind, Donnie Allison got back in front along with Yarborough. The two ran neck and neck over the final laps ahead of Richard Petty, Daryl Waltrip, and A.J. Foyt.

Jeff, a Yarborough fan, and Tim, a Donnie Allison fan, poked fun at each other's drivers as they went back and forth in the lead. Suddenly, Yarborough tried to pass Allison on turn two but was blocked, resulting in an accident. Richard Petty went on to win the race.

"To both of our guys losing," Jeff said, the two men laughing at the antics on the screen that were being replayed. "But also, to what I hope is a great future of NASCAR being televised so everyone can see what a great sport it is!"

The Daytona 500 was first televised on February 18, 1979.

18. The Comic Strip

Jake opened the paper, flipping through the news stories, reading a few, and then stopping at the comics. A new comic appeared that Jake had never seen before called "Doonesbury." This was unlike any comic strip he had ever seen. The first strip had a guy in a football helmet awaiting the arrival of his new college roommate, thinking that a computer was picking the perfect match. When the roommate arrives, it appears the two are mismatched, and the cartoon ends with a comment that there were "still a few bugs in the system."

Each day, Jake looked forward to reading the Doonesbury comic strip. The strip was funny but had far more political commentary than any other cartoon. One strip referred to the Watergate scandal, while others discussed political and social issues of the day. When "quoting" the president, the strip showed just a drawing of the White House as if the words could be heard outside the walls.

Over the years, Jake found that he related strongly to some of the sentiments in the comic strip and began to pay more attention to the political climate. Jeff was excited when the strip won a Pulitzer Prize for editorial cartooning. He began to volunteer for various political candidates whose ideals he believed in, thinking he could be as politically savvy as the characters in his favorite cartoon.

Even when the cartoon creators took a break for several years, Jeff continued to follow their work, traveling to New York to see the Broadway musical based on his favorite characters.

Jeff focused on local and state politics for the remainder of his life, basing some of his talking points on those that resonated with him in the comic strip. He always credited his newfound love of politics to a small, unique comic strip in his local paper in 1970.

Doonesbury, written by Gary Trudeau, appeared for the first time on October 26, 1970.

19. A Dream Realized

The sun shone as Flora walked down the street to the bus stop. This was a new bus stop for her as she was being sent to a different school than she had attended the previous year. Just the year early, the Supreme Court ruled that school districts could bus children into different areas to encourage diversity. As a young black girl, this was going to help Flora tremendously.

Growing up in a poor, primarily ethnic neighborhood, Flora attended the schools closest to her home. Although the teachers were terrific and Flora excelled at academics, they were poorly funded, and the books were usually outdated, hand-me-downs from schools in more affluent areas. Flora had big dreams, and she knew that those dreams would be more brutal to achieve if she did not have an excellent secondary education. The court ruling had allowed Flora to be chosen as one of the students who would now attend a school in a more affluent area.

The bus arrived, and Flora stepped on, happy to see that other students smiled back at her. A few dark-skinned students were sitting throughout the bus, but Flora chose to sit next to a white girl who seemed to smile the brightest at her.

“Hello, I’m Amy,” the girl said, extending her hand.

Flora introduced herself and asked Amy about the school.

“We do a lot of fun things,” Amy told her. “It is not like other schools you may have gone to, as we are encouraged to be individuals. It focuses on getting you ready for a job or for college, whichever is best for you.”

Flora found that what Amy said had been confirmed, the new school offered so much more than her old one. They required her to keep a journal and issued credit for it, plus they placed all students in internships in a corporate setting. Flora was placed in a unique program where she interned at a small local television station, answering mail and helping follow up on leads.

Flora finished her high school education there and studied at a university on a full scholarship. She excelled in college and graduated with a degree in communication. She returned to the local station, where she interned and accepted a position as an educational programmer. Flora always credited the Supreme Court decision with her success in life.

The Swann v. Charlotte-Mecklinburg Board of Education decision by the Supreme Court held that busing was permitted in order to end racial imbalance in schools.

20. A Role Model for Young Girls

The television show captured Nicole's attention immediately. There was a crash landing on an uncharted island with Amazon warriors, women who lived forever in isolation from men. Nicole was fascinated when Hippolyta, the island's queen, sent her daughter, Diana, with the pilot to help him fight the Nazis who would invade the island if they won the war.

Each week, Nicole would tune in to watch as Diana Prince, the name she used as an assistant to the pilot, saved the day, but not as herself. Instead, the bracelets she wore gave her special powers and turned her into Wonder Woman.

The more Nicole watched Diana Prince battled evil as Wonder Woman, the more confidence she felt in herself. Nicole loved that Wonder Woman never seemed to use her beauty to succeed, and she never depended on men to help her. She did not fall in love with every man on the show, including the pilot who took her from Paradise Island. Her magic lasso was only used when she had to use it, relying more on her intelligence and common sense to solve problems.

As Nicole grew up, she often referred to the lessons she learned while watching Wonder Woman. She became independent and used her intelligence to solve problems. Throughout college, Nicole excelled, applying her Diana Prince and Wonder Woman-inspired lessons to her daily life.

Wonder Woman changed how Nicole thought, acted, and proceeded through life. Because she felt Wonder Woman changed her life, she never stopped her children from reading comic books or watching superhero shows or movies. She felt that if they learned as much from the modern versions as she did from old classics, they would do fine in life.

Wonder Woman, starring Lynda Carter, began airing in 1977 and almost immediately became a cult classic.

Welcome to the 80s

1. The Wall Came Tumbling Down

Jacob had long dreamed of a unified Germany, even though his country had been divided since before he was born. The Berlin Wall blocked access between East and West Berlin.
Jacob moved to Berlin right after he finished university, recalling his grandmother's stories about her experiences as a nurse working in Berlin during the war.

When he arrived, he found thousands of people his age protesting against the wall and Soviet control over half the city. Immediately, Jacob joined the *mauerspecte* or "wall woodpeckers" as they began to chip away at the tangible symbol between freedom and oppression.

Jacob remembered when American President Ronald Reagan demanded that the wall be torn down. His words, "Mr. Gorbachev, tear down this wall!" had resonated throughout Germany, and Jacob knew that when the wall fell, it would make his country whole again.

Spending as much time as he could at the wall to protest its existence, Jacob used his hammer and screwdriver, which he had tossed into his backseat when he left home, to knock through concrete sections. He was among those that cheered loudly when their hole in the wall grew large enough that people could cross into the land that had been blocked for many years.

Jacob laughed loudly as the passage between East and West Berlin was opened up so people could pass freely back and forth. He jumped on the wall at one point to celebrate, holding up a glass of champagne he was handed before drinking it down in one swallow. For hours, he simply walked through the hole in the wall, back and forth, enjoying the sense of freedom he never imagined would happen, enjoying the space he had dreamed of.

Jacob knew his actions chipping away at the wall helped free half his country from communist rule. As an older man, Jacob told his grandchildren how he had helped free half of Berlin from tyranny with a hammer and screwdriver.

The Berlin Wall "fell" on November 9, 1989, a symbol of the end of the Cold War.

2. Confidence Booster

Shelly tried to keep her head down as she walked from the school bus stop, hoping that Billie, Jo, and Margie did not see her. For weeks, she had dealt with bullying by the two older girls, and she was unsure what to do about it. She had not mentioned the problem to her parents as she did not want them to go to school and make it worse.

It was a weekend, and Shelly's parents decided to take the family to the movies. They started with dinner at their favorite restaurant in town, and then Shelly, her parents, and her younger brother, Larry, headed to the theater. The movie Karate Kid and Shelly had heard from friends was a perfect movie.

From the minute the film started, Shelly was hooked. She watched as Daniel, the bullied "new kid," learned lessons in martial arts from Mr. Miyagi. She was captivated when Daniel eventually beat the bully in the end. After the movie, Shelly asked her parents if she could take karate lessons. They told her it was an unusual request but agreed, thinking it was good for her to do something physical.

Shelly became devoted to her martial arts instructor, learning to protect herself and gaining more confidence than ever. She knew that the motto of her dojo was not to use karate to hurt someone, but instead, she was taught only to use physical force as a last resort.

Because she had not engaged with the bullies, their actions had gotten stronger and bolder. About a year after she signed up at the dojo, one of them began harassing her at the bus stop, this time coming close to Shelly.

“I am warning you to stop,” Shelly said, finally having enough. As the girls tried to crowd her into the street, she stepped into the grass. Billie Jo, significantly taller and heavier than Shelly, grabbed her arm and attempted to twist it.

In a flash, Shelly had turned her body, gripped Billie Jo’s arm, and flipped her over her shoulder and onto the grass with a thump. Margie just stood there, her eyes wide as Shelly stood over Billie Jo in a crouched stance.

Billie Jo jumped up and reached for Shelly again, but she was not quick enough as Shelly dodged her arm. Shelly spun and kicked Billie Jo’s leg out from under her, and the girl fell again. That was enough to get the message to her, and the bigger girl jumped up, backing away, her eyes wide.

From then on, Shelly never had to deal with bullying again and credited The Karate Kid with her confidence for the rest of her life.

The Karate Kid premiered in 1984, starring Ralph Macchio, Pat Morita, and Elisabeth Shue, creating an interest in martial arts.

3. Time to Get Physical

Walking through the store, Greta leaned on the shopping cart. She was exhausted, and her doctor had just told her she needed to be more active. She was still carrying around the baby weight after the birth of her daughter, and it was starting to cause her problems.

Greta walked through the video section, hoping to find an uplifting movie or something to get her out of her bad mood. There, on a shelf at the end of an aisle, something caught her attention. There was a video cassette with a red and white cover and a photo of a woman in leg warmers and workout clothing. Greta picked up the box labeled *Jane Fonda's Original Workout* to look at it closer.

Jane Fonda isn't a fitness instructor, Greta thought to herself. *She's an actress*. Greta read the back of the box and realized that the actress had ventured into the aerobic exercise business. On a whim, Greta tossed it in the cart. She finished her shopping and headed to pick her daughter up at daycare.

That night after dinner, Greta carried the video into the family room. Her husband was in the garage working on his projects, so Greta figured she would check out the video. There was a half-hour beginner's class, and Greta found the exercises were not challenging. She worked out at the beginner's course that night and then added the workout to her morning routine.

For the next month, she got up an hour earlier to do the beginner workout program, letting her husband and baby sleep. After that month, she moved up to the 60-minute advanced program. People at her office noticed that Greta looked healthier and seemed to have more energy.

Her positive results from doing the workout video encouraged Greta to become more active. The benefits of her new, healthy lifestyle extended to her husband and daughter. Even when Greta became pregnant with her second child, she continued working out as much as possible and, within weeks after her son was born, had returned to her pre-pregnancy weight. As her fitness improved, she became more confident, which stayed with her for the rest of her life, all because she purchased a new workout video.

Jane Fonda released her workout video in 1982, starting a physical fitness craze.

4. Broad Shoulders

It was a beautiful sunny day as Callie walked down the street in her small town. She had just landed her dream job at a local finance office and needed to upgrade her wardrobe to match her new responsibilities. Callie was often timid, hoping to find something that would scream "power" as she entered the male-dominated world of finance.

She glanced in the window of one of the boutiques and saw a beautiful dress on a mannequin. The mannequin's figure looked almost like a "V"; the waist looked nipped in, and the shoulders broad. Callie entered the store and found many versions of the dress, all with padded shoulders. She tried one on and found she loved the look.

"My waist looks so small," she told the salesperson. "And the big shoulders make me feel stronger. That sounds ridiculous, but it makes me feel bigger and more powerful."

Callie purchased several of the dresses and a blazer that also had bigger shoulders. On her first day at work, she was shocked to notice that the men in the office treated her with respect. She initially thought it was just politeness, but she also felt as if she was more apt to speak her mind when wearing the new dress style.

Soon, Callie noticed other women also wearing the padded-shouldered clothing, and it seemed that when they did, the women were taken more seriously. Callie felt that the shoulder pads made the women appear more significant, giving them an air of confidence they had not had before.

As Callie developed more skills, she had more opportunities to move up in the office. Over the years, she purchased many items of clothing with shoulder pads, believing that they improved her look and gave the impression she was talented, capable, and intelligent.

Within ten years, Callie had moved into management, a feat she accredited to purchasing a dress that made her appear more prominent and stronger.

Shoulder pads, although common in the 1930s, made a resurgence in the 1980s, with many women claiming the pads gave them a more angular, defined, and powerful shape.

5. Where Everybody Knows Your Name

Lance dropped his hat on the dining room table, heading down the hall to take a shower and rinse off the smell of grease. Currently working as a line cook in a local diner, Lance spent his days over a greasy cooktop.

Lance heated a frozen dinner and carried it to the living room, where he flipped on the television. A new show was premiering, and he wanted to watch it. The show was about a bar in Boston, not far from where Lance lived, and he was interested to see what it was all about.

The show opens with a song about a place where everybody knows your name. Lance watched as a young woman was left behind by her fiancé, eventually becoming a waitress. He laughed at Norm, Cliff, Sam, Diane, Coach, and Carla. While he was watching, a thought popped into his head.

Last week, on his way home, he saw a sign in the window of a neighborhood bar indicating they were closing. The night after *Cheers* premiered, Lance stopped into the bar to talk to the owner. He asked why they were closing, and the owner told him his kids were not interested in operating it. The owner wanted to retire and decided to shut down the bar.

“What if I took it over?” Lance asked the man. “You stay as owner for a year, and I will rent to own. That way, you get some income, and I can build the bar business.” The owner promised to think about it and asked Lance to stop in the following week.

Lance got through the week at the restaurant but was a bundle of nerves. The more he thought about owning a bar like Cheers, the more excited he became. A week after his talk with the owner, Lance stopped in again.

The owner handed him documents that would eventually make the bar Lance's and explained that the monthly rent he charged Lance was significantly below the income he should expect from the bar. He told Lance the bar was usually busy and that many regulars kept the place humming.

A month later, Lance was behind the bar in his new business. He found the bar very similar to the comedy show he still loved watching. He had his own "Norm," "Cliff," and "Carla." His expertise in commercial kitchens also helped him grow the menu at the bar, attracting even more customers to his friendly neighborhood bar. Lance knew that a television show had changed his life.

Cheers debuted on September 30, 1982.

6. Career and Family

It had been a busy day at the law practice, and Claudia was tired. However, her day was not done when she left the office. Her briefcase was filled with documents she needed to review after she put the children down for the night.

Arriving home, Claudia fixed dinner for her family and supervised baths and bedtimes for her three children. She returned to the family room where her husband, Jake, sat in his recliner, his legal paperwork in front of him.

As Claudia opened her briefcase, she recalled what prompted her to get her law degree. In 1981, she was a young wife, mother, and career woman. Claudia worked as a legal secretary in her husband's law firm, mostly answering phones and typing legal documents. But she yearned for more, knowing she could offer a different perspective at the practice than the men who led the business.

Then, in July, President Ronald Regan appointed the first female Supreme Court Justice, Sandra Day O'Connor, to replace Potter Stewart. This led Claudia to do some research on the nominee. She learned that the proposed justice had difficulty finding a paying job after law school, eventually taking a volunteer job as a deputy county attorney that ultimately led to a small salary equivalent to what a paralegal would earn.

Claudia read that O'Connor had worked as an attorney in Germany. At the same time, her husband served in the military before returning to Arizona, where the nominated justice took five years off to raise her sons. Claudia knew that if a woman could start with such humble beginnings and rise to be assigned to the Supreme Court, she could also achieve her dreams.

With her husband's blessing, Claudia returned to school and earned her law degree in two years. She moved into an office in her husband's firm, where she focused on family law, gaining a reputation for defending women who were victims of domestic violence.

Claudia returned to the documents on her lap, smiling as she recalled how a woman rising to the highest level possible in the legal field was a shining light to women everywhere.

Sandra Day O'Connor was the first woman appointed to the Supreme Court on September 21, 1982, by a vote of 99 to 0.

7. The Story in Pictures

The wedding was beautiful, and the honeymoon relaxing. Michael and Jennifer had returned home a few days before and were settling into a routine. They were excited to see photos from the wedding.

Just the year before, disposable cameras became available in stores. Because they had grown in popularity so quickly, Michael and Jennifer decided to place a disposable camera on each table and encouraged guests to take photos. Michael had dropped off the 20 cameras at the drugstore the day after they arrived home, planning to pick them up at the end of the week.

While away on their honeymoon, Michael and Jennifer laughed about some photos They had seen their guests taking. Michael's brother, Mark, and Jennifer's sister, Lisa, were notorious pranksters, so they imagined they had taken some pretty funny photos. As the bride and groom walked around talking to guests at the reception, Michael recalled taking quite a few pictures with their guests.

Michael brought the packs of photos home that week, and the two eagerly opened each package, flipping through the hundreds of pictures from their wedding. They laughed at some of the crazy faces and weird angles of some of the photos. Jennifer's eyes welled with tears at one taken as she and her father danced, the tears in her father's eyes evident as he looked down at his daughter.

Some photos were blurry and out of focus, but it did not matter to Michael and Jennifer. They looked them over multiple times, laughing each time they saw some in particular. Six months later, when Jennifer's grandmother passed away suddenly, Jennifer was thrilled to have good photos of her from the wedding, many of which she framed to remember her Grandma.

Many years later, when they both had lost their parents, Jennifer and Michael returned to those wedding photos. Many included other guests that were no longer living. Jennifer and Michael were always thankful that the disposable cameras were available on the day they married, simply for the memories those cameras brought to them decades later.

The disposable camera made its appearance in 1986, with the first manufactured by Fujifilm.

8. The Boat to Freedom

Only 11 years old, Maria was frightened. Her mother, father, and brother stood in the holding camp where a government car had dropped them off. They had been there a week before they were taken to the Port of Mariel, where the entire family was on a shrimp boat.

As a child, Maria knew that the boat was overcrowded, but she also knew that her parents had promised her and her brother a better life in America. It would take more than a day to reach their new home. The boat left the dock, and they began the journey to the southern coast of Florida.

The trip was not pleasant. Waves as high as two-story buildings battered the little boat. Maria felt that the ocean water could not have been darker, the waves scarier. She held on to her mother tightly while her father gripped her younger brother, the four of them struggling to remain in the boat. The boat's captain told horror stories of how other ships had capsized, and many people had to be rescued on this journey.

Over 24 hours later, Maria and her family docked in Key West. It was still dark, but the sun started peering over the horizon. Maria and her brother were excited to see a Coca-Cola machine at the end of the dock, a sign they had arrived in the land of freedom. She was shocked to see the people on the pier who were there to help them.

The family made their way up the coast of Florida to a small town just 30 miles north of Miami but a world away from the problems that some of those who traveled from Cuba faced. Her parents immediately began working toward citizenship, and several years later, all four of them took the oath as American citizens.

The Valdez family thrived in their new home. Eventually, Maria and her brother attended college, which would never have been possible in their native Cuba. The Mariel Boat Lift carried Maria and her family into a new world of promise.

Fidel Castro allowed thousands of Cuban refugees to seek asylum in the United States in 1980.

9. Real Men Do Eat Quiche

The business trip was going well, and Rob was meeting one of his colleagues for breakfast to finalize a deal. This was the first time Rob had represented his company at a conference, and he was excited that he could lock down a deal so quickly.

Dan was already in the restaurant when Rob arrived. The two men shook hands and settled in at the table. The waitress brought them menus and filled their coffee cups. They spread out paperwork on the table before glancing at the menu.

When the waitress returned, Rob ordered the quiche Lorraine and was surprised when Dan looked at him strangely. Dan ordered the breakfast special of eggs, bacon, hashbrowns, and toast. When the waitress walked away, Rob reached for the paperwork, but Dan stopped him.

“So, you have not read the book yet,” Dan said, smiling at Rob. “The *Real Men Don’t Eat Quiche* book?” Rob shook his head.

Dan explained that it was a tongue-in-cheek book that poked fun at masculinity stereotypes and the title had been a catch-all for what made men more masculine. Rob laughed at the insinuation that because he ate quiche, he was not manly.

"Oh, it is a really funny book," Dan said as they looked through the contracts. After all the documents were signed and tucked away in briefcases, the topic returned to things the book said real men don't do.

According to Dan, the book referred to men who eat quiche as the type of man who focuses more on trends than being masculine. This led them to discuss masculinity and what men do to appear more muscular. They both laughed after deciding that eating quiche had nothing to do with masculinity since most quiche was created from bacon and eggs.

The two men parted ways, laughing about how an author tried to make a simple breakfast dish into something it wasn't — a symbol of gender identity. The discussion led to them becoming close friends, and they often enjoyed quiche together from that point forward.

Real Men Don't Eat Quiche, a book by Bruce Feirstein, was published in 1982.

10. I Want My MTV

The college dorm was busy as Waylon headed down the hallway. It was midterms, and more students were in common areas, studying or working together on projects. Waylon found his way to the quad's center, where a grouping of chairs surrounded a large television screen. He needed a break from studying, so he'd headed down to hang out with friends.

He heard music as he entered the seating area and glanced at the television. There was a video of Van Halen with David Lee Roth singing “Jump” as Waylon plopped into one of the chairs. The song ended, and Wham’s “Careless Whisper” began playing.

“Whoa, what is this channel?” Waylon asked. Another classmate told him it was MTV, and they only showed music videos. Waylon was sucked into the videos, enjoying the antics of Devo with their flowerpot hats, followed by Peter Gabriel’s artistic music interpretations.

From that day on, Waylon would take some time in the common areas of the dorm to watch a few videos, seeing bands he had never heard of, and gaining a love of music that crossed genres. He ignored the critics who said it was a passing phase as he felt the music video was the way of the future.

Over the years, Waylon developed a love of music that helped him through many of life’s ups and downs. When he and his wife married, they danced to “Against All Odds” by Phil Collins as it was a video they both loved. When his children were young, Waylon would sing songs from iconic videos, like Dire Straits’ “Money for Nothing,” sometimes dancing around the same way the artists did in the video. As they got older, his dancing often embarrassed his children, leading him to do it more often.

When his father died, Waylon requested that Cyndi Lauper’s “Time After Time” be played at the funeral. The music he recalled from the early days of MTV stayed with him for the rest of his life. He would always identify the artistic exposure of music that had never been seen before and often watch those videos over the years as a reminder of his college years.

MTV premiered on August 1, 1981, with a broadcast of "Video Killed the Radio Star" by the Buggles.

11. Check the Cabbage Patch

Gloria stood in line at the store. Her fingers crossed that this time she would successfully get the one thing her daughter wanted for Christmas, a Cabbage Patch Doll. Last night, she heard that Montgomery Ward was receiving a shipment of the hard-to-get dolls, so she and her sister, Becky, stood in a line that seemed to wrap entirely around the building.

The store manager stood at the door, allowing only four people inside at a time. There were about 50 people ahead of Gloria and Becky, but they shuffled forward, hoping that this time they would successfully get a doll for Gloria's daughter, Heather, and Becky's daughter, Noreen.

Finally, the two women entered the store and walked over to the display. There were about 30 dolls piled up on the shelf, but the two women were not allowed to pick their own. A store employee handed them a box with a doll in it and instructed them to take it to the register.

Heather ran into her parents' room on Christmas morning and jumped on the bed.

"Get up!" she cried, her three-year-old body moving like a bouncing ball. "I want to see if Santa came!"

Gloria made Heather wash her face and brush her teeth before heading downstairs. When they arrived in the living room, Josh handed Gloria a cup of coffee as she sat beneath the tree and began handing out gifts. As she gave Heather the last package, she could see the disappointment on the child's face because she had not gotten the doll she wanted. The previous package was far too small to be a Cabbage Patch.

Gloria winked at Josh as she stood and walked into the kitchen, telling Heather to come to help her with breakfast. The little girl liked breaking eggs into pancake batter. She wandered behind her mother into the kitchen, her head down initially.

Sitting in Heather's old high chair, was a Cabbage Patch Doll, her little pile of paperwork on the tray in front of her. Heather squealed and ran to the chair, snatching up the doll. Gloria and Josh laughed as Heather hugged the doll tight. Josh picked up the paperwork.

"Oh, there is a pledge you have to make," he told Heather. "Hold up your hand." Heather raised her hand and looked at her father.

Josh read from the paper, telling Heather to repeat what he said.

"I promise to love my Cabbage Patch Kid with all my heart," Josh read with his daughter repeating after him. "I promise to be a good and kind parent. I will always remember how special my Cabbage Patch is to me."

From then on, Heather and her Cabbage Patch, Loralee, were inseparable.

The Cabbage Patch craze began in the winter of 1983.

12. The Missed Birthday

Turning 16 only happens once, and Kelly was excited that her birthday was in a few weeks. Not only was her 16th birthday coming up soon, but her older sister's wedding also was the weekend before, so there was a lot of excitement in the house.

In preparation for the wedding, Kelly's grandparents were arriving that day, another thing to look forward to as Kelly adored her grandparents. She expected they would bring her gifts for her birthday; as was a tradition in their family, a special dinner would be planned.

To Kelly's surprise, when her grandparents arrived, they mentioned nothing about her birthday but seemed focused entirely on the wedding. Since her birthday was a week after the wedding, Kelly just assumed there would be more focus on her once the wedding was over.

The wedding day arrived, and it was as beautiful as everyone anticipated. Her sister and her new husband left on their honeymoon the next day. Kelly knew everyone would talk about plans for her birthday once her sister went, but no one said a word. Her grandparents left the following day.

Kelly was heartbroken as she thought there would be a big celebration for her 16th birthday. She remembered that her sister's 16th birthday included a nice dinner with friends and family, but no one had even asked Kelly what she wanted to do.

The morning of her birthday, no one said anything to her. There was no special breakfast, and no one asked her where she wanted dinner. It was as if her parents had forgotten entirely what day it was. Later that afternoon, Kelly's mother asked if she wanted to ride to the country club, still saying nothing about Kelly's birthday. Kelly agreed, just to have something to do.

Her mother reminded her she needed to dress nicely for the club, so Kelly put on one of her summer dresses. Her father was playing golf at the club, so Kelly figured they would just have a regular dinner there.

Kelly walked into the country club's restaurant behind her mother and jumped as she heard "surprise" from everyone in the room. All her friends and family were standing there, the room decorated with balloons and streamers. Kelly grinned widely as her parents came over to her.

"I thought you forgot," Kelly said, hugging them.

"We could never forget the day you were born," her mother said. "We just knew with the wedding, you were not getting much attention, so we planned this celebration for you."

The movie, "16 Candles," was released in 1984 and told the story of a girl turning 16 whose parents forget her birthday due to her sister's wedding.

13. USA for Africa

Growing up in Ethiopia, Menelek remembered what changed his life. In June 1985, a plane carrying food, medicine, and clothing arrived, bringing hope to those starving in his country. This food and clothing helped Menelek grow strong and healthy, eventually immigrating to the United States.

The food and clothing came from an unlikely source, Menelek learned when he arrived in the United States. In March 1985, the song “We Are the World” was released. The song featured dozens of famous musicians who came together to record a song that would be used to raise funds for humanitarian efforts in Africa.

Those humanitarian efforts led Menelek to succeed as he was in contact with missionaries who provided him with an education. The only member of his family to graduate from high school and attend university. Menelek knew his fortune could be made in the country that had provided him with the assistance he needed to succeed.

Once he arrived in the United States, he could watch a video of the song that changed his life. He saw Stevie Wonder, Huey Lewis, Michael Jackson, Diana Ross, and more singing about the need to help the world. He also knew he wanted to help as many people as possible.

Menelek completed medical school in the United States and eventually became a doctor. He often traveled back to his homeland, offering free medical services to people in Ethiopia. He never forgot that it was this type of humanitarian aid that helped him achieve his own goals.

Over the years, Menelek learned that the recording that gave him hope as a starving child raised millions to help benefit people around the world who were suffering. He also learned that the proceeds assisted agriculture projects, and taught water and fishing management while helping to reforest areas of his homeland.

Menelek would forever be grateful for the many artists who came together to record a song. Since then, similar projects have been organized to raise funds and awareness, and the proceeds have continued to provide life-saving assistance.

"We Are the World," a charity single recorded by the USA for Africa in 1985, sold more than 20 million copies.

14. News at Night

His long night shift over, Kevin headed to his car, his jacket tossed over his shoulder. It was a warm night, actually more generous than when Kevin had arrived at work that afternoon. Heading home at midnight was never pleasant, but his plant operated 24 hours a day, so that meant shift work.

Kevin pulled into his driveway about 20 minutes later. He thought to himself that at least there was very little traffic in their small town at this time of night on a Sunday. He dropped his keys on the table in the hallway and headed to the kitchen. His wife had left his dinner in the fridge with a note signed with a heart. Kevin popped it into the microwave and grabbed a beer. The ping of the microwave was loud in the quiet kitchen, and he wondered, as he did every night he worked shift work, how it did not wake up the kids.

Grabbing a fork and knife, Kevin headed into the living room and put the plate on a small table in front of his recliner. He turned on the television and began searching through the channels. Suddenly, he stopped on a new medium he had never seen before.

It looked like a news channel with a man and woman at the desk. The screen switched to a man interviewing President Jimmy Carter.

As he ate his dinner, Kevin was fascinated as he watched the news reporters ask John B. Anderson debate questions, and then he listened to his responses. Then there was a recorded segment of Ronald Reagan and President Carter answering the questions. Kevin was fascinated as he watched, thinking this was one of the most unique news programs he had ever seen.

Starting that night, Kevin came home from working the late shift, grabbed his dinner, and watched the new news station. His coworkers were shocked when Kevin began talking about things that happened in the news. He became a follower of *Moneyline*, developing a solid understanding of finance and economics. The more he watched the show, the more intrigued he was with those subjects.

One day, while getting ready for work, he saw an advertisement for a local community college. Kevin picked up the phone and called the number on the screen. A young woman on the other end set up an appointment for him to come in and discuss his options.

A week later, Kevin was registered for economics classes at the college. Two years later, he graduated with an associate degree in the subject. With his wife's encouragement, he transferred to a four-year university, graduating with a bachelor's in economics. His shift work days were over as he accepted an economic advisor position with the city.

CNN, the first 24-hour news network, aired its first episode on June 1, 1980.

15. A Farewell Speech

After dinner, the family gathered in the living room around the television. For the last time, President Ronald Reagan would speak to the country. Erin and Sean settled onto the sofa while Cora and Ben plopped on the floor. The children were not thrilled that they were required to watch the speech, but their parents believed it would instil in them a sense of civic duty and pride.

"This is the 34th time I will speak to you from the Oval Office and the last," President Reagan began. "We've been together eight years now, and soon it'll be time for me to go. But before I do, I wanted to share some thoughts, some of which I've been saving for a long time."

The president continued, stating what an honor it was to hold the office, also expressing thanks from his wife, Nancy. Ben sat up straighter as the president continued, telling a story about a refugee who called a sailor a "freedom man."

Ben looked at his father, whose eyes were glued to the television.

"Dad, is this why you are in the Army?" Ben asked.

"It sure is, son," his father responded. "Our job is to protect the freedoms the president is talking about. Today, the world is at peace because we have worked hard to convince those who have been fighting to stop. Kind of like when you and your sister get in a fight, Mom and I have to convince you to stop."

"I was raised to believe you had to pay your way for the blessings bestowed on you," the president said. "I was happy with my career in the entertainment world, but I ultimately went into politics because I wanted to protect something precious."

After the speech ended, that quote stuck with Ben. He also felt like he wanted to protect something precious. Throughout his high school career, his mind returned to that quote. He had known from a young age he wanted to follow in his father's footsteps but he decided to go to college and enter the military as an officer. He rose to the highest level in the military and, after retiring, entered the political arena, serving as a state senator for many years. He told anyone who asked why he entered politics that it was all because of a farewell speech by a president.

President Ronald Reagan gave his farewell speech in 1989 after serving two terms as President of the United States.

16. Living Life to the Fullest

The movie ended, and Paul stood to leave the theater, his mind racing. Although the characters in the film had gone overboard with their pranks and skipped school, the film speaks directly to Paul.

Growing up in a small town, Paul never felt like he could expand his horizons. When the main character in the movie repeatedly said that a person should believe in themselves, Paul realized he never had. As the film continued, Paul began to see how confidence could take someone's place.

Never a rule breaker, Paul knew he could not go as far as the group of friends in the film. After seeing the movie, Paul began to relax more and began to see what rules were meant to be broken. He never did anything that would result in his grades being lowered or things that would get him in serious trouble, but he broke minor rules, like coming home a bit later than he was supposed to or not doing a chore quickly.

At college, Paul felt he had a better grip on what he needed to do. Many of his fellow first-year students spent too much time partying, enjoying the freedom they did not have at home. Paul's mindset was different. He still wanted parties and hanging out with his friends, but he incorporated his fun into his education.

After graduating college, Paul knew he wanted his career to include fun. He applied for a position as the director of youth programs at a local community center. The job was the perfect blend of fun and business, precisely what Paul needed. Every day he went to work, Paul thought back to *Ferris Bueller's Day Off*, the movie that had changed his life.

Ferris Bueller's Day Off premiered on June 11, 1986.

17. Technology Arrives

"You are not going to believe what they are installing in our office," Shane said, coming in the door from work. "We are all getting computers on our desks, an Apple II. We have a weeklong training on it next week."

His wife smiled as she stirred something on the stove, turning her cheek so Shane could kiss her.

“Computers have been around for a long time,” Brenda said. “What is the issue?

Shane pulled a beer from the refrigerator and leaned against the counter.

“This is different,” he said. “We will all have a computer at our desk. Before, we just had them here and there.”

When Shane arrived at work the next day, the new computer was sitting at the end of his desk. It had a standard typewriter keyboard, two small boxes with slots above it, and a screen that looked like a small television. That week, during training, Shane learned how to use the machine and found that he enjoyed using it.

Shane found that he could complete tasks faster, giving him time to focus on things he had put aside due to time constraints. He also found that he liked figuring out why the computer was not doing what he expected it to do.

A few weeks later, Shane went to his boss and asked about available positions involving more computer work. He found his work was far more manageable with the machine and thought he would like to learn how to maintain and troubleshoot them.

Not long after that conversation, Shane was sent for extensive training on the new computers. He learned how to troubleshoot issues with the machines, common problems that may arise as the computers were used, and advanced technology related to computers. He was assigned to the newly formed technology department when he returned to the office.

His wife often reminded him about his hesitation to use the machines when they were first placed in the office. She reminded him each time he was promoted in the technology department, eventually becoming head of the department. The Apple II that landed on his desk in 1985 was the springboard to an entire career for Shane. By the time he retired, technology had changed significantly, coming a long way from the clunky Apple II that began his new job.

Although released in 1977, the Apple II did not become the best-selling PC until 1985, when 2.1 million were sold.

18. The Wedding of the Century

Holly was beyond excited as she entered St. Paul's Cathedral. She had tucked her invitation in her small purse after showing it to the guard at the entrance. She found a seat near the cathedral's center, adjusting her hat slightly.

She could not believe she had received an invitation to the wedding of Prince Charles and Lady Diana Spencer. Holly and Diana had worked together at a local school, becoming friends, but not close friends. She was thrilled when the invitation arrived, knowing this wedding would be stunning.

Over the past few weeks, the press had been relentless with coverage of the royal nuptials, talking about this being the first wedding of an heir to the throne since Prince Charles' mother, Queen Elizabeth, married many years ago. Today had been declared a national holiday in Britain, and the streets were filled with people trying to glimpse the couple. Holly smiled as she sat inside the cathedral while many others were standing outside, all packed together on the sidewalks.

The crowd began cheering, and Holly realized the royal family must be arriving. Later, she learned that Charles arrived in an antique carriage while Diana arrived in a glass coach with her father. The orchestra began playing “Trumpet Voluntary,”, and everyone in the cathedral stood, turning to look at the bride as she entered.

Diana was stunning in her ivory gown with lace, sequins, and pearls. The train was incredibly long. Holly thought it must be about 30 feet long as it trailed halfway down the aisle after Diana arrived at the altar.

During the vows, everyone, including Holly, giggled as Diana incorrectly said Charles’ name and when Charles made a mistake in his vows. As the couple left the church, the crowd clapped and followed behind them. They were headed to Buckingham Palace for a wedding breakfast.

Holly waited outside with the crowd to see the traditional kiss on the balcony, then headed inside to celebrate her friend's wedding, the Princess of Wales.

Prince Charles and Lady Diana Spencer married on July 29, 1981, a wedding that many considered a fairy tale.

19. The Yuppie Escape

Josie sat in the sunroom of her large home, sipping coffee she and her husband, Lance, had imported from Columbia, where they had taken their last vacation. She looked over the swimming pool and gardens, wondering why she felt so restless.

Lance, a corporate attorney, was advancing in his firm rapidly, likely making partner the following year. Josie, a commercial real estate broker, was equally successful, allowing them to purchase the Spanish-style historic home near Hollywood. The house was tucked into a neighborhood of similar homes, all older but with stunning landscaping. Josie and Lance had a wine cellar full of expensive bottles, none of which they needed to "save for a special occasion."

Harriet, the cleaning lady, poked her head in the sunroom to ask about a particular article of clothing as she was doing laundry. Josie responded absently, still wondering what was making her so restless. She picked up the magazine by her side, thinking it might change her mood. Inside the magazine was a story about living simply, removing all the extras in life to have a quieter, calmer life.

That night at dinner, Josie told Lance about the article, explaining that it hit home for her as she had recently struggled with restlessness. To her surprise, he agreed.

"I love what I do, but I would also love to get out of this rat race," he told Josie.

For weeks, the couple talked about what it would be like to walk away simply. Could they sell the home they adored, quit their jobs, and live simply? Lance began to research the option of opening his private firm.

Soon, an opportunity presented itself as if it was meant to be when their friends came for dinner one evening. They talked about how they had just taken jobs in London but could not take their two German Shepherds due to quarantine rules. They planned to return to the United States in a few years and were looking for someone to live in their home, rent-free, to care for the dogs.

The next day, Lance and Josie told them they would do it. They immediately put their home up for sale and stored items they did not want to part with or items with sentimental value. The rest were sold with the house. They moved to their friends' home in a small beach town in California, where they cared for the dogs. Lance commuted to his corporate job for about six months before opening his practice in the beach town. Josie opened her real estate firm in the local area, keeping it as small as possible to provide personalized service.

Within one year, Josie and Lance had given up the young urban professional lifestyle, or "yuppie" as it was called, to live simply, frugally, and happily. The pressure to be at the top was gone, and they often talked about that magazine article that had started it all.

In 1984, Dan Rottenberg called young urban professionals with considerable affluence "yuppies," but by 1987, many of these professionals were downsizing to simplify their lives.

20. Home at Last

Blindfolded, Barry knew he was outside but had no idea where the kidnappers had taken him. They had been told to pack their things, but he was unsure why. All around him, his fellow hostages were screaming, their fear palpable. The kidnappers were also calling as the group was pushed forward and ushered onto a bus. Barry could hear crying and knew that others felt as he did, that they would be executed.

The bus stopped, and they were pushed to the door. As Barry stepped off the bus, his blindfold was snatched from his face, and he blinked in the bright lights. He realized they were at the airport, and confusion set in as the group was shoved toward a waiting airplane. They sat on the runway for what felt like hours before they took off. The hostages looked at each other in a daze before someone spoke.

"Are we going home?" Kathryn asked, her voice shaky. A soldier standing at the back of the plane confirmed that the hostages had been freed and were on their way to the United States. Someone opened a bottle of champagne, and glasses were passed around. Barry was too dazed to drink, despite his jubilation that he was free. After so many days in captivity, he was worried about what life would be like.

First, the plane took them to Germany, where they spent a few days in the hospital. All Barry wanted was to see his family.

Finally, the plane landed at a small airport in New York, and as they stepped from the plane, they were greeted with cheers from a large crowd. A yellow carpet led them into the airport, where Barry saw his wife, Barbara, and his two children, Alexander and Ariana. They ran towards him, and the four embraced, all of them crying.

The next few days were a blur for Barry. He met former President Jimmy Carter and the current President Ronald Reagan, who announced during his inaugural address that Barry and his colleagues were on their way home. He attended a service at St. Patrick's Cathedral, where they received a standing ovation. The prayers at Temple Emanu-El before the ticker tape parade in their honor seemed surreal.

Barry was ready for his life to return to normal after spending 444 days as a hostage in a foreign country, and he never took freedom for granted again.

On November 4, 1979, Iranian students stormed the U.S. embassy in Tehran, taking hostages who were not released until January 1981.

Welcome to the 90s

1. The Toy That Talked

Mary entered her daughter Hailey's room and looked at the row of furry, big-eyed toys on her dresser. As soon as they felt her presence, the creatures began to blink their eyes, and one of them chirped. Mary smiled at the Furbies before waking her daughter up for school.

"Good morning, dear," Mary said, lightly tapping Hailey's shoulder. The child rolled over and opened her eyes, rubbing the sleep out of them. "Remember, you have to take care of your Furbies before you go to school."

Hailey hopped out of bed and walked to the dresser, and Mary watched as her daughter patted each one on the head and spoke to it. The little furry creatures sometimes responded, mostly in gibberish that Mary didn't understand, but a few responded with what sounded like actual words.

"Are you teaching them to talk, Hailey?" Mary asked her daughter. Hailey responded that Furbies could learn the language of the people who owned them. She explained that it takes a bit but that her Furbies were beginning to understand the words she said.

Hailey then began pressing the tongues of her Furbies, and Mary laughed as she watched the little creatures "eat" as Hailey cooed at them to finish their breakfast. Mary left the room to finish breakfast and let Hailey get dressed.

When her daughter came downstairs, Mary asked her how the Furbies were. Hailey told her mother she had petted them all again, and now they were all asleep. Hailey ate her breakfast, and Mary walked with her to the bus stop and waited until she got on the school bus.

That afternoon, Mary entered Hailey's room to gather the child's dirty laundry. She glanced at the Furbies and laughed at the little creatures standing in a line with their eyes closed.

It is so lovely that Hailey has found these little toys, Mary thought to herself as she carried the laundry downstairs. *At least she has some friends in the house since she has no siblings*.

For many years, Hailey took care of her Furbies. All of them learned to speak English, and she often played music to dance with them. Even as a teen, Hailey occasionally closed herself in her room and listened to music. Mary could hear her singing and the little furry creatures moving on the dresser. She would smile, knowing that the Furbies were dancing to Hailey's music.

Furbies, one of the first interactive toys, were released in 1998 by Tiger Electronics.

2. In the Palm of Your Hand

Elizabeth walked by the electronics store and stopped when a device in the window caught her eye. The little sign in front called it a Palm Pilot with a price tag of $399. Intrigued, Elizabeth walked into the store.

"It is the latest in handheld devices, far better than a pager," the salesman said as she looked at the device. "It can connect to your computer so you can sync your address book, your calendar, and even keep track of expenses.

As a busy executive, Elizabeth always sought ways to streamline daily activities. She decided to purchase the device and see how it worked. When she got home, she set everything up and installed the device's software on her computer.

The next day, she carried the little device to the office. An email arrived regarding a meeting with one of her colleagues to discuss a marketing plan. Elizabeth remembered her new little device and decided to test it. She pulled it out of her purse, pulled out the tiny stylus that came with it, and began tapping on the screen.

Within seconds, she had scheduled the meeting on her calendar. Later that day, after having lunch with a client, Elizabeth decided to see how it worked to track expenses. She was able to enter the cost of the lunch and set a reminder to add it to her expense account. When she got to the office, Elizabeth plugged the device into her computer and smiled as all the information she had entered loaded into her laptop.

At the next board meeting, Elizabeth showed her colleagues the new device. She suggested the company purchase them for the entire board to streamline and organize their company. The commission agreed, and Palm Pilots were in the hands of the board of directors within a week.

From then on, executives could be seen with their Palm Pilots in their hands, tapping on the tiny screen and organizing their day. The Palm Pilots were a feature in Elizabeth's company for almost ten years until the advent of portable phones that offered better options. Elizabeth never forgot how a stroll by an electronics store helped her company become more efficient.

Palm Pilots were released in 1996, and by 1998, 30 million had been sold.

3. The Boys in the Band

Finding their seats, Ashley and Laura settled in, both of them quivering with excitement to see their favorite band finally. The two girls had woken up early, chosen special outfits, and spent hours on their hair and makeup just in case a band member noticed them.

The two girls danced to the opening band's music even though they were not familiar with the band called The Perfect Gentlemen. Then, about a half hour after the opening act finished, they heard the music they had been waiting for.
New Kids on the Block took the stage singing "Call It What You Want." Ashley, Laura, and everyone around them jumped up to their feet and began screaming.

"Donnie looks so handsome!" Ashley cried as her idol danced and sang on the stage.

"Look at Jordan!" Laura screamed, her hands waving in the air.

Laura, Ashley, and the crowd danced to two lesser-known songs, "My Favorite Girl" and "Valentine Girl." When they launched into "You Got It," the crowd went wild. Ashley and Laura stood in their seats, waving their arms and dancing.

The boys on the stage danced and sang, going through their song set as the crowd went wild. Ashley and Laura had never screamed or danced so much. Suddenly, a man in a suit walked over to the end of their row and got their attention. He said the two had been chosen to go backstage after the concert to meet the band in person.

The band finished their concert with their famous song, “Hangin' Tough.” As the rest of the crowd made their way to the exit, Ashley and Laura made their way backstage with about seven others. The man in the suit guided them to a door next to the stage.

Behind the stage, there seemed to be hundreds of people, all moving quickly to roll up wires, gather microphones, and simply get everything ready to be loaded for the next concert. The man walked them to another door and opened it. Standing there were Jordan, Joey, Donnie, Jonathan, and Danny.

Most of the other fans chosen from the audience seemed to freeze as they saw their favourite band members up close. Donnie broke the ice, walking over and shaking the hand of the young man who was the first in line. The fans moved into the room, where they mingled with the band.

“We love doing this,” Jordan told Ashley. “Just going on the road and entertaining the fans, that's amazing.”

Donnie and Ashley talked for a few minutes, and he gave her some advice she held close for the rest of her life.

“Every single moment is a moment to cherish,” he told her. “Cherish each one. Cherish each second. Life is a gift, don't waste it.”

During the 1990s, “boy bands” were extremely popular, like New Kids on the Block, New Edition, NSYNC, Backstreet Boys.

4. A Video Game in Your Hand

Jason sat at his computer, wasting time until he could shut down for the day. Despite working from home, he tried to keep set hours, signing into his computer by 8 AM and not signing off until 5, except for the hour he took for lunch. He decided to visit an online auction account that had recently become so popular.

As he was browsing the website, an item popped up that Jason had utterly forgotten about. There, available for bid, was a Game Boy, one of the original versions still in its box and mint condition. Just seeing the small machine took Jason back to his childhood when he had begged his parents for one of the handheld consoles.

“You are most certainly allowed to have one,” he remembered his father saying. “But you have to earn the money for it yourself.” At 15, Jason initially resented the comment, wondering how on Earth he could raise $100 to purchase this engineering marvel.

Every day that summer, Jason rode to work with his mother and spent his day putting documents in alphabetical order before heading to the file room to slide them into manila folders. He lost count of the number of papercuts he earned as he tackled the mounds of paper that seemed to grow each day. At the end of the week, his mother handed him cash which he tucked into an envelope in his room.

Finally, after the fourth week in her office, Jason counted his cash and discovered he had earned enough to buy the Game Boy. He rushed to the dining room and asked if his mother would stop at the department store that afternoon to buy the machine. She agreed, and that night, Jason finally held his coveted prize. Looking back now, Jason smiled, realizing that the device was challenging to use. It had no light on the screen, and, after dark, it was almost impossible to play unless Jason lay on his bed backward. The game angled toward the hallway door with the light from the living room flickering into his room.

Now an adult, Jason could not resist, and he placed a bid. A few days later, he discovered he was the highest bidder and paid the balance immediately. Within a week, he held the console in his hand, two accompanying cartridges on the desk before him. Simply having that Game Boy in his hand carried him back to the summer of his 15th year, and he could not wait to lose himself in it again.

Released in 1989, the Game Boy became extremely popular during the 1990s.

5. A Trip to the Mall

Leslie and Rhonda were giggling with excitement as they hopped in the car. Leaving their small children with their husbands for the day, the two women were heading out of the city to attend the opening of what had been billed as the largest mall in the country. They could not wait to visit what had to be more like a city than a shopping mall with more than 300 stores.

"I heard there was even an amusement park inside!" Leslie exclaimed as Rhonda backed her car out of the driveway. The two women chatted about what they may see when they arrived at the mall, but nothing could have prepared them as they pulled into the parking lot. Thousands of people stood waiting to get inside, lined up outside glass doors under a giant red, white, and blue star logo.

People had their faces pressed against the glass, trying to glimpse the interior as mall employees fought to hold them back. The building was huge, and Leslie's eyes grew large as they rode around to find a place to park. Finally, after what seemed like hours, the two women found a space some distance from the mall, but they were so excited they did not mind the walk.

They got in a line that seemed to wrap around the building just as the doors opened. People began to stream inside, Leslie and Rhonda included. Once inside, they learned that the mall had four main sections, each with a different theme. The amusement park in the center, Knott's Camp Snoopy, featured the Charles Schultz "Peanuts" comic strip characters, and the women were thrilled when they caught a glimpse of the comic creator himself standing in the park.

Wandering through the giant mall, Leslie and Rhonda visited hundreds of stores, sometimes just to see what the store was about, and made a few purchases for their families. Rhonda found some adorable dresses for her minor daughter, while Leslie bought some new blue jeans for her two boys.

Despite concerns that it would not be much of a success, the Mall of America lived up to its name on opening day.

The Mall of America, a project in the making for 20 years, opened its doors on August 1, 1992.

6. The Surprise Winner

With the coveted ticket in her hand, Gretchen made her way to her seats above the ice rink at the Olympic Games. Since she was a young girl, Gretchen dreamed of watching figure skating at the Olympics. Her career in foreign service had finally allowed her to achieve that dream. When it was announced that the Olympic games would be held in Nagano, Japan, Gretchen knew she would pay any price to get seats in the ice arena. The fact that she was there to see the women's finals was just the icing on the cake.

An American living abroad, Gretchen was well aware that two United States skaters were favored, and she fully expected to be present when Michelle Kwan won Olympic gold at this competition. She was also excited to see a little-known skater, Tara Lipinski, who had seemed to climb to fame over the past few years.

Gretchen had been following the ice-skating competition, watching Michelle win the short program and Tara came in second. Sitting in her seat in the arena, Gretchen was sure the two women would take gold and silver, believing that Michelle would stand on the gold podium while the lesser-known Tara would take the silver.

Sitting through the programs, Gretchen was thrilled to watch as the female skaters twirled and jumped their way across the ice. Michelle's performance was stunning, and Gretchen was shocked when the judges awarded her high marks for presentation but lower technical marks.

When Tara took the ice, however, the mood in the arena shifted dramatically. Her youth seemed to permeate the room, and the crowd leaned forward in anticipation of her performance. Tara did not disappoint. The people in the stands could almost feel the young girl's excitement as she skated in the free skate competition. It was almost like she was just enjoying herself on the ice and was unaware that she was fighting for Olympic gold.

Her double, triple loops almost brought the house down as she landed them flawlessly. Gretchen thought that her ending combination was almost perfect, her hands pressed to her mouth as she leaned forward, almost holding her breath. When Tara finished, clearly breathless, her smile was radiant, and Gretchen and the rest of the arena leapt to her feet, applauding. Flowers rained down on the ice as Tara took her bows.

At that point Gretchen realized she had just witnessed a very young woman make Olympic history, and tears streamed down her face as she watched Tara Lipinski accept the gold medal.

In 1998, Tara Lipinski was the surprising Gold Medal winner at the Olympic Games in Japan, the youngest to ever win gold.

7. Be Like Mike

The basketball court was empty as Steven bounced the ball across the concrete. It was early morning, and he had just enough time to throw a few hoops before heading back inside his apartment to shower for work. Although he knew he would never reach his idol's level, watching the man on the court encouraged Steven to try to play better.

Once a week, Steven joined other young 20-somethings in a high school gymnasium, playing the sport he loved. He wasn't the best player, but the one thing he had learned studying his idol was that he did not have to be the best. All he needed to do was his best, to give it everything he had on the court.

One thing that Steven had realized since he'd started following the pro player he had come to admire so much was that he could apply what he learned to anything he attempted. After college, he accepted a position at a local advertising agency. Spending time on the basketball court had taught Steven that the only person holding him back was himself.

His idol taught him to learn every aspect of the game, which didn't just apply to basketball. Steven spent his days learning every part of the company, gaining the confidence to reach his goals faster than he had anticipated. He also learned to trust the people he worked with, just as his idol trusted his teammates to succeed. In reading up on the man he had come to respect so much, he learned that he never took credit for a team's success. Instead, he gave credit to those who surrounded him as well.

Steven also developed the ability to succeed under pressure. The tighter the deadline, the more he shined. He became the person others came to when a deadline was looming, and they were stuck on a project. Steven could dig into the project's meat and narrow down the focus so the deadline was less intimidating, helping others reach their own goals.

Steven thought back to his recent promotion as he threw the basketball through the hoop at the court outside his apartment. He now headed an entire group of advertising executives, providing them with the same guidance he learned from his idol. He checked his watch and realized it was time to head inside for a shower. He stood back at the three-point line and tossed the ball again, grinning as it made the satisfying swoosh through the hoop.

Steven grabbed the ball and headed inside, sending silent thanks to Michael Jordan, the basketball player he had never met but who had given him the confidence to succeed in everything he did.

Michael Jordan led the Chicago Bulls to an NBA Championship in 1991, encouraging many people to "be like Mike."

8. An Online Lifeline

Lester sat in his office, staring at the balance sheet his accountant had sent over the day before. The numbers were dismal, and he didn't know what to do. The business his grandfather began 60 years earlier was struggling, and Lester was running out of options. The company sold industrial machine parts and had gone from making $50 million in sales to less than $8 million. The company had already laid off half its workforce, with many more layoffs in sight if something didn't change.

Their area had been hit hard by the recession, and Lester knew it was not just his own company that struggled. Many large industries had closed their doors, and joblessness was at an all-time high. He was trying his best not to lay off any more of his faithful staff, but his balance sheet didn't lie. His accountant's predictions in the note attached to the financial documents were even more frightening.

"You are projected to drop to less than $1 million in sales in the next 18 months, and that figure will continue to drop if your business model does not change. If things stay as they are, this company will close its doors in less than three years."

Just then, Lester's office door opened, and his chief operating officer, Alan, walked in, with a grin.

"I think I have a solution to our problems," Alan said, dropping a pile of paper on Lester's desk. Lester looked at the documents and saw an inventory list. Reading down the list, he recognized a lot of small, inexpensive items that they had determined did not have a significant enough profit margin to advertise. Alan suggested they put the employees they had left to work clearing out the unwanted items by selling them on a new online platform called eBay. Lester agreed, and they put a group of staff members to work, organizing, photographing, and listing the items for sale.

The plan was an immediate hit, and everything in the pile they had considered dead inventory was gone, increasing revenue to $50,000 monthly. Pivoting their marketing strategy, Lester and Alan decided not to publish their catalogs that year, a savings of $75,000 each, and to simply market everything through eBay.

Within two years, revenue had returned to the $50 million the company earned before the recession. Lester was able to hire back all the laid-off employees plus more, and today, the company still has a solid online presence.

eBay, one of the first online auction websites, launched in 1995.

9. The Skater Jeans

Never fitting in had become customary for Sean, although when he was sailing around on his skateboard, he felt invincible. It was lunchtime at his high school, and he was sitting outside the cafeteria at a table alone. Movement near him caught his eye, and he turned to see a few guys with paint cans working on a wall.

Sean turned and watched as the graffiti artists worked quickly, and he saw that they appeared to be outlining letters. After the letters JNCO were visible, the artists filled the design in with color, adding what looked like waves, fields, trees, and other images. As quickly as they arrived, the artists were gone.

That afternoon, Sean was at the local skate park when he saw one of his fellow skateboarders enter wearing a pair of jeans with extensive legs. Soon after, a few people he did not recognize entered the park and began talking to the other skaters. Sean walked over to see what they were discussing. The men handed each skater a plastic bag with what appeared to be a pair of jeans. They told them that they were free samples for them to try.

Sean took them home and pulled on the jeans. They were unlike any other pair of jeans he ever wore. His legs were so wide they covered his shoes, and his waist sat low on his hips. He was sold immediately and could not wait to wear them to the skatepark.

When he got there a few days later, he saw many skaters wearing the new style of jeans. The pockets of the jeans were bottomless and felt more like a pair of shorts than jeans since the legs didn't bind around the ankle.

The skaters began chatting about the jeans, mentioning the murals they had seen around town and commenting that they liked the jeans, mainly because their parents hated them. When the school began to suggest they were unsafe, Sean and his friends decided the jeans were the perfect anti-establishment message.

When he reached adulthood, Sean looked back and laughed at the pictures of him wearing jeans with a pantleg at least three or four feet wide, but he also smiled at the memories it brought him of his life as a rebellious skater.

JNCO jeans debuted in 1993 and quickly became a hot seller among anti-establishment teenagers.

10. Gotta Catch Them All

The small yellow creature on the screen spun quickly before a puff of smoke changed it to a different-looking creature. Lorena grinned, realizing she had just evolved one Pokemon into another character. Lorena loved the video game, spending her time battling other trainers and defeating the champion. She took on the elite four and tried to keep the evil villains from dominating the world.

One of the reasons Lorena loved the game is that it seemed to mirror real life to her. It was impossible to beat every trainer, which meant sometimes you had to face defeat, just like in life. She realized that things would not always go smoothly, but she could achieve almost anything as long as she did her best and bounced back from setbacks.

The other thing she loved about evolving from a Charmander to a Charmelon and then a Charizard was that it taught her to be prepared for anything. The abilities of each Pokemon evolution could involve different strategies, which meant she had to be ready in case the other trainer used something against her she wasn't expecting.

Lorena used many of the lessons she learned playing Pokemon in real life, building a sense of perseverance and strength many others in her workplace did not have. In her mind, the video game was the key to her success in everything she attempted.

Pokemon was released in the United States in 1996 and soon became extremely popular, which inspired cartoons, movies, and more created based on the characters.

11. You Can Search for It

The rain was bad enough, but when the thunder and lightning began, Alicia knew she was in trouble. Sitting in her dorm room, she once again thought how stupid she was to have waited until the last minute to finish her term paper. With the stormy weather, there was no way she would be able to walk to the library, and all of her friends with cars were unavailable.

Alicia sat looking dejectedly at the computer on the desk in her room. She had a few reference items stored on the computer but knew that it was not near what she needed to meet the requirements of the paper. The door to her room opened, and her roommate, Nina, walked in.

"Are you still working on that paper?" Nina said, plopping on her bed.

"I wish," Alicia said. "With this storm, I can't get to the library to finish my research, and this paper is due tomorrow. I have no idea how I am going to do this. Do you think the professor checks references? Maybe I can just make them up."

"You have Professor Domakin," Nina said. "Not a chance. He is a stickler for good research. You know he will at least check a few of them. But I may have a solution for you." Nina hopped from the bed and walked over to the computer.

After pressing a few keys, the university internet page popped up. This was a relatively new addition to their college's resources for students, and Alicia had not done much with it other than look up her grades or talk to her professors. Suddenly, a strange-looking screen with colorful letters spelling "Google" appeared. Under it, she read the words out loud, "Search the web using Google" and "Index contains 25 million pages (soon to be much bigger)." There was even a section to enter an email to sign up for updates and a place to go to the Stanford Linux Search.

"Okay, what is the topic?" Nina asked. Alicia told her, and she entered the information in the white box under the search comment. Within seconds, a list appeared, all with titles related to Alicia's term paper. Nina instructed her to click on one of them. When Alicia did so, a scholarly article appeared with information Alicia could use.

"What is this?" Alicia asked.

"I learned about it in one of my tech classes. It is a new thing called a search engine," Nina said, returning to her bed. "Now, get that paper done so we can go to the pub."

That night, the world opened up to Alicia. She finished her term paper using the articles and citations she found on Google and discovered that there was a world of information available now at her fingertips.

Google launched in academia in 1995 and to the rest of the world in 1998.

12. Learning Can Be Fun

It was after dinner, and Craig sat at the dining room table, his books spread in front of him. He hated school, and homework was the worst part of it. His sister, the outstanding student, had finished her homework when she got home and was now in her room playing.

"I think you are just trying too hard," his mother said as she wandered by. "Maybe try to figure out a way to make learning fun." She dropped a book on the table and walked away.

On the front of the book was a woman with curly red hair, and a bus that appeared to be flying behind her. Despite not being a good student, Craig loved to read, so he carried the book to his room once he was done with his homework.

The book transformed him. In the book, the teacher with the frizzy hair took her class on a fantastic ride on the flying bus into space.

Her dress had rocket ships on it. While flying around the atmosphere, the teacher provided details about everything they saw, and Craig remembered some of it from his science class that week.

From that point on, he was hooked on the books. Each time he asked, his mother would bring him a new one, and Craig started to better understand some of the subjects he was learning. Each book opened his eyes more and more, and he began to understand how learning could be fun.

Craig’s grades improved, and he started to get his homework done right after school like his sister. He knew that if he got his work done, he could disappear into his room and read more about the teacher's adventures and her magic bus. Each book focused on a different subject, exposing him to many other things. He was surprised when he started to grasp some complicated issues in his classes because he had read about them in his books.

For the rest of his life, Craig credited the books in the *Magic School Bus* series with helping him develop a lifelong love of learning.

The Magic School Bus was released in September 1994 and has been credited with teaching children many different subjects in a fun way.

13. The Hedgehog

The little blue hedgehog on the screen was adorable, Paula thought. Her father had just brought the new game home for her game system, which was already proving interesting. The little hedgehog had a little bit of an attitude, something that Paula wished she had as well.

After moving to a new school, Paula had few friends and spent most of her free time in her room playing on her video game console. She played a multitude of games, like *Batman* and *ESwat.* She loved those games, but her new favorite was the little blue hedgehog who was impatient, just like Paula.

The new school was difficult for her, and there was a group of kids who bullied her relentlessly. Paula was an introvert who preferred art to sports and didn't fit in well at the new school. Every day, she would escape to her room and her tiny blue hedgehog who was saving his friends and running toward them rather than running away from problems. The little hedgehog transported Paula to another world, giving her a different reality than the one she was living in.

The more Paula played the game, the more she realized she could be like the little hedgehog. She could fight for what was right, and stand up to the bad guys, even the bullies in her school. One morning, the bullies began their verbal assault against Paula, and she'd had enough. She walked to the principal's office and demanded to see him.

Once in his office, Paula told him everything she had been dealing with. A group of kids had been attacking her, threatening her life, and even stalking her at home. After being insulted today, Paula summoned the strength of her little hedgehog friend and decided to do something about it.

The next day, the children bullying Paula were not in school. She learned that she had not been the only one they were terrorizing, and the school had chosen to expel them after learning some horrible things they were doing. Paula never saw them again as her family moved soon after, and she changed schools.

Paula did not doubt that *Sonic the Hedgehog* helped her grow the confidence to stand up to the evildoers in her school and take a stand.

Sonic the Hedgehog was released in 1991 and grew into a multi-game franchise throughout the decade and beyond.

14. The Wizarding World

Getting lost in a book was not unusual for Michael. His mother knew when she could not find him. He was likely curled up somewhere reading. Books transported Michael away from his everyday life and into another world. When his mother handed him a thick book with pink and blue letters on the cover, he had no idea reading it would change his life forever.

Inside that book, a world unfolded that, although the ultimate fantasy, gave Michael a sense that it was based on his own life. Inside was the story of a young boy who had powers he never knew he had, sent to a school that he never knew existed through a magic train station.

Michael saw endless possibilities as he read about Harry and his friends. The strong friendships created almost from the very first page of the book reminded Michael of his small circle of friends.

Still, it also provided him with a look into the future instead of being constantly focused on the past as was typical for Michael.

Although the main character did not have a wonderful childhood, something Michael did have, his adventures in the book reminded Michael that no matter where he went in the world, there was no place like home. For Harry, the home ended up being Hogwarts or wherever his friends were. Michael began to realize how much the book impacted him as he grew up.

As Michael moved on to other books in the series, he began to talk about what he was reading with his friends. They sat around talking about what the last Horcrux might be or why the author constantly placed a twinkle in Dumbledore's eyes. Michael started searching for information about the series online, discovering fan fiction, podcasts, and more that allowed him to talk with other fans about how important this book was to his life.

Throughout his high school years, Michael returned to the lessons he learned while reading a book series about a child wizard. Even in college, he joined clubs related to books. After earning his degree, Michael started a career as an editor at a publishing company, where he realized the most important lesson. Just because a book focused on magic, was written by someone unknown and seemed to be unusual in the commercial world, that book could still be a viable commodity and it molded the way he looked at books from that point forward.

Harry Potter and the Sorcerer's Stone was released in 1997, followed by Harry Potter and the Chamber of Secrets in 1998 and Harry Potter and the Prisoner of Azkaban in 1999.

15. College Tuition

The application was on her desk, but Robin was unsure she even needed to fill it out. Her family didn't have the money for college, and she had filled out more scholarship applications than she could count. A few had come through, but only for small amounts. She didn't have any idea how she was going to cover the cost of school.

Her mother walked into the room and saw the look on her daughter's face. She asked what was wrong.

"I just don't know how I can pay for school," Robin said. "Why send in an application if there is no way for me to pay for it."

Robin was surprised when her mother simply smiled and left the room. About an hour later, she returned with several clear boxes. Inside, there were small stuffed animals. Robin's mother placed them on the desk.

"Beanie Babies, Mom? Really?" Robin asked, rolling her eyes. "How are these going to pay for my college?" Robin's mother told her to look them up online. Robin turned on her computer and headed to eBay, plugging in the name of the first bear, Wallace.

When the screen came to life, Robin could not believe her eyes. A bear precisely like the one her mother owned was for sale. What was equally surprising was there were two other listings for the bear too. Actually, her mother had three Wallace bears. The current bid for the entire set was $75,000. She typed in "Bubbles," the little striped fish in the fourth box on the desk, which had listings on eBay with bids at $40,000. Robin calculated the total and was excited to discover that these four stuffed toys could pay for her college education.

Robin realized there were two more stuffed toys on her desk, a rabbit named Hippity and an adorable platypus named Patti. Looking both of those up, she found each one had bids for $25,000, bringing the total amount possible for selling these toys to $165,000, and it could be more if the proposals kept rising. She turned and looked at her mother.

"Yes, I have been watching the value of these," her mother told her. "I knew that one day we could sell them and raise money for something important. List them for sale, and let's see what happens."

That afternoon, Robin photographed and placed the six toys on the auction site. Immediately, people began bidding on the stuffed toys. By the time her auctions ended, Robin had enough money for college and additional funds to help her mother.

Beanie Babies were introduced in 1993 and became one of the hottest collectibles around.

16. Music That Changed Lives

She had never heard this type of music before, but from the first note, she realized this would change her life. Charlita couldn't help but sway to the sound, but the lyrics spoke to her. A young black woman living alone in the big city, Charlita was struggling like many others were, young, poor, and ignored by many industries. This music she was hearing for the first time not only spoke to her as part of her culture but also as someone young who was constantly underestimated by those who were older.

After work, Charlita began to frequent clubs that played this type of music. She bought CDs created by Lil Wayne, 2Pac, Public Enemy, and more. She watched videos of these artists who had skin like hers and who were making a name for themselves, but they were not hiding the culture they came from. This empowered Charlita more than anything that had ever happened in her life.

Often, Charlita heard others talk about how hip-hop wasn't music, just a bunch of people speaking words to a beat. She disagreed as she felt the words they were saying were extremely powerful. These songs didn't sugarcoat what was happening in big cities. Instead, the songs took on things like violence and drug use head-on, discouraging those listening from falling into those traps.

One day, while listening to the radio at work, an older hip-hop song came on, and it got Charlita's attention. Run-D.M.C.'s music "Pause" began to play. Charlita had never heard the song before, which opened with lines about drug use and how it destroyed the black community. She had been exposed to drug abuse when a friend became addicted when she was in high school; this hit close to home for Charlita.

A few days later, Charlita was walking home and passed a drug rehabilitation center she had paid little attention to before. Something told her to go inside, and she walked up to the reception desk. The song she had heard a few days earlier made Charlita think about where she wanted to be in life. Because the song made her feel about her high school friend, who was now clean, Charlita realized she wanted to do something to help others have the success her friend had achieved.

She asked the receptionist what steps she would need to take to become a drug and alcohol counselor. The receptionist went into the back office and brought out a manager who sat down with Charlita and outlined what she needed to do. Less than a year later, Charlita walked into the same drug rehabilitation center as a certified counselor, ready to start her first day of work.

In 1997, hip-hop, a genre of music that celebrated black culture, became very popular, giving rise to stars like Tupac Shakur, Notorius B.I.G., Public Enemy, and more.

17. The End of the World

It was 1999, and Marina was at her desk at work. The year was just another one for her, so she tapped away at her computer as she did every day. Marina was entering information in the company database, adding names, addresses, phone numbers, and the dates customers registered with her company. The date field required her to enter six digits: the month, day, and two-digit year.

Marina entered "99" all day for the year that new customers joined or existing companies renewed. Then, one day while taking a break, she noticed an email from one of her bosses. The subject of the email was "The Millennium Bug." Intrigued, Marina opened the email.

Inside, her boss explained that the company was reviewing its computer programs as there was the potential for a crisis. Because their systems were set up with a two-digit year, it was possible that, on January 1, 2000, all of their data could be lost or damaged when the computers reset the year to 1900. This problem was potentially going to cost the company millions to address.

When Marina got home that evening, she turned on the news and learned that the email was just the tip of the iceberg. She knew that the government was very concerned about what they called "Y2K" as much of what they did was computerized. The problem was so widespread the president created a particular webpage to address it, as there were concerns about planes being unable to fly or more devastating implications, such as nuclear weapons being released due to the date issue.

At work, Marina helped the technical department address the Y2K concerns. She was instructed that a new four-digit year field would be added and that she would have to go in and add the two additional digits to everyone's account. Every day, when Marina finished her new data entry, she went customer by customer to make sure the year was correct.

On January 1, 2000, however, there were relatively no incidents. A few countries had plane or train scheduling problems. There was no Y2K crisis, and Marina believed it was because she and others had prepared for the potential disaster.

Throughout 1999, the world was concerned about Y2K, believing that the date fields that contained only two digits instead of four could result in multiple disasters, none of which occurred.

18. The Sunken Ship

For the third night in a row, Jade was in line at the theater, and just by looking at how long the line was, she felt she would be disappointed again. Of all her friends, she was the only one who had not seen *The Titanic.* Her work schedule was wild and it was sometimes impossible to have a social life.

The line moved slowly, and the woman in front of her turned to Jade.

“This is the fourth time I have tried to see this movie,” the woman said.

“It is my third,” Jade told her. “All my friends have seen it and keep telling me that I HAVE to see it.”

Jade explained to the woman that she had been a Titanic buff since she learned about the tragedy in middle school.

“I think I have read every single book about it,” Jade told the woman. “I don’t know why, but the entire story fascinates me. Maybe I was a passenger in a past life.”

The lady laughed.

“Me, too!” she exclaimed. “I have seen every movie about it, too, but I understand this one is one of the best. I think it is supposed to tell the story from the perspective of the rich people onboard as well as the poor people who were on the ship.”

Jade nodded her head as the line moved up again. Jade began to get her hopes up as only a few people were in line in front of her.

“I must also say that Leonardo DiCaprio is quite a cutie,” the woman said to Jade as she took another step toward the ticket booth. Jade laughed.

“He certainly is!” Jade said. The woman walked up to the ticket booth and requested a ticket. Jade’s heart jumped as the ticket clerk took the woman’s cash and handed her a key. The woman turned and gave her a thumbs-up before heading into the theater.

Jade walked up to the window, her hands shaking. She asked for a ticket to *Titanic,* and when the woman handed her the key, Jade almost cried. She headed into the theater, stopping at the concession stand for popcorn and a drink before going inside. When she walked down the aisle, she saw her friend from the line who clapped when she saw Jade.

“This seat is empty. Come sit here,” the lady said, and Jade took the seat. She could hardly contain her excitement as previews for upcoming movies flashed on the screen. She had a feeling this would be one of the most memorable films of her life.

The wreck of The Titanic was discovered in 1985, but learning about the tragedy in our history gained even more popularity when James Cameron released his movie in 1997.

19. Opening the Windows

Jackson was excited to try the new operating system he had just purchased for his home computer. Windows 95 was touted as one of his generation's most innovative programs, and he wanted to see what the hoopla was about.

He arrived home and opened the package, loading the floppy disks into his computer's disk drive and copying the software to his laptop. He then pressed the buttons and waited as the new system loaded. At that point, the messages on his screen advised him to shut down and restart the computer, which he did. When the screen came to life again, Jackson's eyes popped open.

Gone were the MS-DOS prompts and boxy-looking graphics. Instead, his screen had little windows with descriptions that made sense. At the bottom of the screen was the Start menu which Jackson clicked on. It opened up a list of everything on his computer, and Jackson was hooked.

As a computer game player, the ability to move around in the system quickly was one of the best features for Jackson. He could click in and out of programs, go to his email, and search the web from the central computer screen, something he could never do before. Jackson realized he would no longer need to rely on his tech-savvy friends to help him with his computer at home. Windows 95 was simple and easy to use.

The next day at work, Jackson went into the office of the technology manager and told him about the new software. He learned that the new system would be installed on all the computers in the office, but the manager was concerned that people would be unable to learn the new way of navigating the system. Jackson offered to learn the system and be the point of contact for the staff.

Over the next few months, Jackson developed a keen understanding of Windows 95, spending his day moving around the system and learning every thing he could about it. When the technology department released the new approach to the entire company, it was Jackson who people were referred to when they had an issue. Jackson found himself answering questions regularly, helping his coworkers understand this new system.

Over time, his knowledge led him to be put in charge of the help desk at his office, and as newer versions of Windows were released, he became the expert throughout the company, all because he uploaded the program at home when it was new.

Windows was officially released in 1985 but did not become mainstream until 1995.

20. The Rachel

Chloe felt like she was in a rut and was looking for a way to spice things up. She felt like all she did was go to work and come home with no social life. Chloe had just broken up with a boyfriend and felt she needed to shake things up.

It was time for a haircut, so she made an appointment with a new salon in town, one known to be edgy and unique. Karl, her stylist, sat her in the chair and fluffed her hair.

"I think I have the perfect cut for you," he said. Reaching behind him, he grabbed a magazine with a young woman on the cover. Her hair was thick but cut in layers, ending at her shoulders. The layers flipped out from her face in light waves.

"I like it!" Chloe said, smiling. "Let's do it." Before the cut, Chloe's hair was long, hanging below her shoulders, straight, and parted in the middle. It was thick, but she rarely bothered to do much with it. Chloe felt the new haircut would feel lighter and start her on a path to a less boring life.

When Karl was done, he spun the chair around, and Chloe's eyes grew big when she saw her reflection. She loved the new cut as it framed her face and made her feel much more energetic. After leaving the salon, she decided not to go straight home. Instead, she stopped at a local pub, found a place at the bar, and ordered a glass of wine.

"Hey, what are you doing here?" She turned to see who was talking to her. It was Sam, her friend, Bonnie's brother.

"Oh, my goodness! Sam!" Chloe said, jumping out of the chair and hugging Sam. "I have not seen you in what, four years!" Sam laughed.

"I almost didn't even recognize you," he said, taking the stool beside her and ordering a beer. "You look so different," Chloe admitted she had just come from getting a new haircut, so that might be the change.

Sam shook his head.

"No, you seem so confident," he said, sipping his beer. "The kid I remember hanging out with my sister was so shy." Chloe smiled but was shocked. She did feel more confident with the new haircut, which seemed crazy, but something was different about her. Without stopping, she asked Sam if he wanted to join her for dinner.

He grinned at her.

“That would be great,” he said. “Do you want to eat here or go somewhere a little quieter?”

Chloe suggested they walk around the corner to a little Italian restaurant she liked so they could catch up. Sam insisted on paying the bar tab, and they headed down the street. They were seated at a table for two in a corner of the restaurant, where they started by catching up on what was happening with Bonnie, their parents, and Chloe’s brother, Nick.

Before they knew it, the restaurant was empty, and they were the only ones at the table. Chloe was shocked to realize they had been there for almost four hours. She gave Sam her phone number, and they promised to get together again.

When Chloe got to work the next day, she received many compliments on her new hairstyle, but the best part of the day was when she received a call from Sam asking if she would like to meet for dinner again that night. She agreed, and from that night on, they were inseparable. A year later, Sam got down on one knee at the Italian restaurant where they had their first date. Of course, Chloe said yes.

This year, they will celebrate their 20th wedding anniversary, and Chloe has credited their relationship to the “Rachel” haircut she got on a whim.

The Rachel was a haircut made popular by Jennifer Aniston in the show Friends.

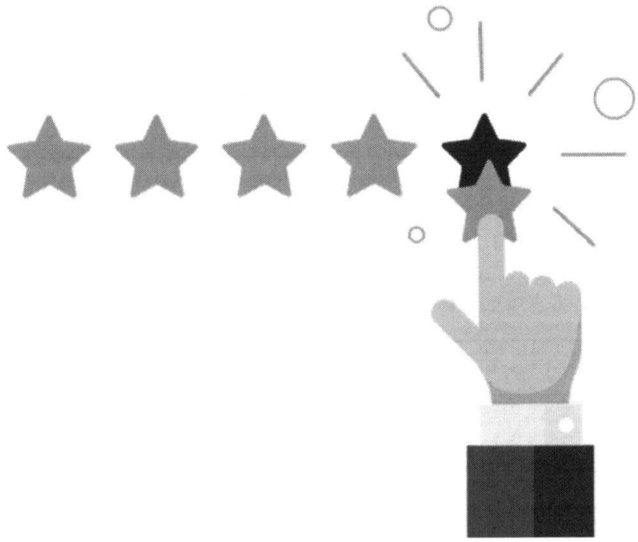

If you have any comments, suggestions, or questions about this book, please email contact.wegamedia@gmail.com. With your help, we can make future editions even better. We would also greatly appreciate a review on Amazon.

Keep Your Mind Young

Printed in Great Britain
by Amazon

35241179R00097